Keep Going

A Story of Resilience and Faith

Sarah Christy

BALBOA
PRESS
A DIVISION OF HAY HOUSE

Balboa Press books may be ordered through booksellers or by contacting:

Balboa Press
A Division of Hay House
1663 Liberty Drive
Bloomington, IN 47403
www.balboapress.com
1 (877) 407-4847

Print information available on the last page.

ISBN: 978-1-9822-1602-3 (sc)
ISBN: 978-1-9822-1604-7 (hc)
ISBN: 978-1-9822-1603-0 (e)

Library of Congress Control Number: 2018913313

Balboa Press rev. date: 11/13/2018

CONTENTS

INTRODUCTION

Alone we can do so little,
Together we can do so much.
—Helen Keller

Merriam-Webster defines *resilience* as "the ability to become strong, healthy, or successful again after something bad happens" and faith as a "belief and trust in and loyalty to God."

My hope for you, the reader, is to be encouraged. While my sister, Marylee, and I faced tragedies and challenges in our lives, we did not quit. From our father's death when we were only eleven and twelve, to our lives today, we have felt the hope of a better tomorrow. Through our ongoing belief in God and his guidance to sustain us, we have been able to move forward. Being confronted by untimely deaths, war, divorce, and major illness, we somehow recognized these tragedies would not define us. We were able to rise and embrace opportunities while engaging in the joy of living.

This recovery would have not been possible without many people's support, encouragement, prayers, and good wishes. A special acknowledgment belongs to our mother, Mary Herrick, who has always been our cheerleader. At the age of one hundred, she continues to stay engaged in our lives and encourages us every day. She modeled for us the philosophy of "keep going even when it's hard." She said, "If you cannot do anything about it, let it go and move on." She nurtured our creativity, giving us a view that life is full of possibilities. We thank all whose stories we tell.

The working title of this book was *Two Sisters and a Little Boy*. Rod's energy and influence as the "*Little Boy*" are at the center of this book. I, his mother, and Marylee, his aunt, have felt the presence of his energy and spirit as we have worked in creating this story. We are forever thankful for him.

We want to emphasize this story has a cast of many who joined us on our journey. God moved people in and out of our lives at times when we needed them most. His promptings led us on this journey. To God be the glory!

Sarah Christy and Marylee Nunley

CHAPTER 1

Two Sisters

Small town girls keep their feet planted firmly on
the ground—no matter where they end up.
—Anonymous

A black-and-white picture of two little girls in matching outfits sits on my desk. Taken in the 1950s, the picture reminds me of the joy of a childhood shared with my sister and the amazing lives we enjoy today. Many of the years were in tandem, each of us pursuing our own interests and creating our own lives. Always knowing we are connected, supportive, and available. Today, we, two small-town girls, are part of a national nonprofit organization that serves hundreds stroke survivors and their caregivers across the country. This is our story.

Our childhood world revolved around our small midwestern hometown. We rarely traveled away from it. Most people made their living farming or working in strip coal mining. I was the second child and the first daughter, arriving in 1946—the beginning of the baby boom. My father had been stationed in the Aleutian Islands in Alaska while serving in World War II when my older brother, Rodney, was born. My father was able to be present for my arrival and babyhood. Taking after his side of the family, I felt a special connection with him and was proud to be named for his mother.

My mother would repeat the poem:

> Monday's child is fair of face, Tuesday's child is
> full of grace, Wednesday's child is full of woe,
> Thursday's child has far to go,
> Friday's child is loving and giving, Saturday's child
> works hard for its living,
> But a child that is born on the Sabbath day is fair
> and wise and good and gay.

I was born on a Sunday, the Sabbath. My heart would swell with happiness when I heard the saying. My sister, Marylee, was born a short fifteen months later. Because I was so young, I have no recollection of her arrival. We shared a bedroom, were known as "the girls," and were inseparable.

This was an era of peace and prosperity. The United States had won the war. The soldiers were home. Our small town felt safe and friendly. We enjoyed a childhood filled with love, nurturing acceptance, and encouragement. We experienced the security of two loving parents, a brother, and many extended family members, which included our maternal grandparents who lived within walking distance of our home. This was our whole world.

Although we were close in age, we were encouraged to develop our individual personalities. School was easy for both of us. We enjoyed the freedom to play imaginatively. Marylee and I loved to write, stage, and act in skits of our own concoction. We had a box of "show clothes." I recall the thrill when our mother would discard a pair of high heels or a particularly beautiful dress—and we could add it to our show clothes box.

Building tree houses, riding bikes, and playing kick the can at dusk were some of our best summer memories. When we had a neighborhood baseball game, my brother always sent me to the outfield to catch fly balls. He wanted me to take the game seriously. I did not. After a few minutes, I would become bored, getting in trouble with my brother for doing cartwheels instead of watching for the ball coming my way.

As a child, I loved books. Going to the public library was magical to me. I vividly remember turning ten and being allowed to get my own library card instead of using my mother's card. I was thrilled to know I could check out any book in the building. I discovered a row of biographies on a shelf, all bound in the same orange cover, and read every one of them in order. One summer, my friend Randy and I created our own library in his basement. We borrowed books from friends and neighbors to stock our inventory. I do not recall anyone coming and checking out a book. I imagine soon we were off to another adventure like building a tree house.

Our father worked one full-time job and another part-time job. Often, he wasn't home in the evening. After the dishes were done and the kitchen was cleaned up, our mother would play with us. I have many memories of creating skits, acting out nursery rhymes, playing charades, spin the pan, and different board games. We were one of the last families in town to get a television. I don't think we had missed having one, but once it was installed, we enjoyed watching it. A new tradition was added to our week. On Sunday nights, we were allowed eat in front of the television while watching *Lassie*. We often enjoyed special local treats of kitchen-cooked potato chips and glazed doughnuts from Betty Ann Bakery.

We were surrounded by extended family. Our mother had six siblings, and our father had four. Holidays meant family gatherings. Easter and Thanksgiving were celebrated with our father's family. Thanksgiving dinner was at Aunt Vi's. Uncle Howard, a businessman, had purchased hair clippers and taught himself to cut hair. All the boys lined up and got haircuts. In the spring, we would go to Aunt Dot and Uncle Phil's farm. I have a less-than-pleasant memory of chasing pigs in the field.

The Fourth of July, Christmas, and New Year's Day celebrations were with our mother's family. Fourth of July meant fireworks at Grandma and Grandpa's. In the 1950s, all the family chipped in to purchase fireworks and would light them in an open field. Big firework extravaganzas that we are familiar with today were not part of life in our small town. I recall the long wait for the sky to get dark and our family's annual treat of ice cream floats. The ice cream went into the glass first, then the orange soda was poured in, and the orange foam would rise to the top to be slurped first.

On Christmas morning, we would arise to see what Santa had left for us. Unwrapping the rest of the gifts had to wait until my grandparents arrived. The adults ate a big breakfast and drank "gallons" of coffee before we got to open the gifts. My grandparents didn't have a television. On New Year's Day, my uncle would bring them to our house to watch the parades on our television.

The biggest family highlight for Rodney, Marylee, and me was the annual family reunion. Uncle Merrill and Aunt Franny hosted the reunion on their land in the country. It was always held in July when the cousins from both Texas and Boston would be visiting. Thinking of the family reunions of my childhood, I remember a day of pure joy with all of the kids playing, unrestrained from the daily rules. We would play hide-and-seek, weave crowns of clover, and enjoy the freedom of running free. There was an old-fashioned pump where we got drinks of cool water using the communal tin cup that hung from its side. We would use the pump to wash off our feet, allowing the cold water to splash over them.

The uncles would set up a card table and play cards under the big maple tree. My mustached grandpa, unable to see the cards, would sit in a chair near them, puffing on his pipe and listening to the play and conversation.

When it was time for dinner, we would find the table loaded with family favorites. Aunt Mildred would make a fruit salad containing whipped cream. In order to keep it cool, she brought a large cut-glass bowl, filled it with ice, and then nestled a second glass bowl that held the salad in the ice. I viewed this as very clever and beautiful. A large crock filled with lemonade was always set out with a metal dipper and a large block of ice floating in it to keep it cool. We would dip our own drinks.

The only family trip we took was in 1952 when our family of five when to Chicago to visit Aunt Alice (my mother's sister) and Uncle Dan. I recall three exciting experiences while there: visiting Lincoln Park Zoo, Riverview Amusement Park, and Buckingham Fountain in Grant Park. Visiting a big city was exciting for our small-town family. I had never seen a skyscraper, a body of water as big as Lake Michigan, or the vast number of people and cars. One night, we went to Grant Park to see Buckingham Fountain, one of the largest in the world. The night was magical, watching the twenty-minute show of colored lights and music as the water shot into the air making the fountain a spectacular sight.

Both Marylee and I have distinct memories of going to Riverview Park, a popular amusement park. I was paired with Aunt Alice in the bumper cars. She had no idea how to drive. Everybody was bumping into us, and even though I was only six, I was ready to grab the wheel and take over. Four-year-old Marylee recalls riding on the merry-go-round. She was entranced with beautiful painted horses going up and down. Nine-year-old Rodney was fascinated by the psychic sideshow. There was a lady dressed in white flowing clothes on the stage with a man walking around the audience, offering the opportunity to ask a question for a fee. Uncle Dan was trying to figure out how the lady on the stage could get the "psychic information" from the man. In an effort to deduce this, he paid for our mother to ask a question of the woman dressed in white on the stage who mysteriously provided answers.

At Lincoln Park Zoo, we were exposed to animals we had never seen. Marylee was captivated by the monkeys and the chimpanzees. She recalls how her fascination with the primates was beyond description. These feelings have stayed with her and she still finds them magical. As she watched them, she wondered what was going on in their little minds. *Could they think like a little girl? And wouldn't it be fun to swing and jump like them?* The following Christmas,

Marylee received a Phoebe B. Beebe doll, the chimpanzee that was on the 1950s *Today Show* with Dave Garroway. Phoebe was her very own buddy to play with—to talk to—her new lifelong friend.

Another important part of our lives was the Christian faith. Both of our parents came from families of faith and were members of the local Methodist church. We grew up regularly attending church. Marylee and I liked Sunday school and participated in church activities. Even as a child, I felt drawn to faith and a belief in God's presence.

Life dramatically changed on a cold January morning in 1959 when I awoke to quiet voices coming from the living room. I was confused and frightened and wondered why there were people in our house so early in the morning. Our mother came into the bedroom and broke the news to Marylee and me that our father had been killed in a car accident. A crushing blow for two young girls, ages eleven and twelve. The next few days passed in a blur of friends of friends and relatives and the rituals that surround a death. I remember Uncle Howard packing my father's clothes in the trunk of his car and taking them from the house. I recall the smell of funeral flowers, the hushed voices, and strange foods donated by friends and relatives—all things that reminded me that my life had forever changed.

No longer were we happy girls heading into adolescence; we were two girls lost and sad. At the funeral, I looked up at a picture of Jesus and thought: *He will be my Father now.* That was the moment I committed myself to living a life filled with a Christian calling. Marylee remembers feeling like our daddy might be walking with Jesus. Since Jesus could see us, maybe our daddy could too.

Each of us learned to walk our way through a difficult time of life. We lived in a family and era when grief was ignored and pushing through the pain was private. However, that didn't mean that Marylee and I were exempt for our own challenges of grief. We both remember the early days when going to school was difficult.

We thought people would treat us differently because we no longer had a dad.

For Marylee, security was found in her Phoebe B. Beebe chimpanzee doll. She felt lost and lonely much of the time—except when she had Phoebe B. Beebe with her. She spent hours playing and imagining Phoebe as her closest confidante. I remember struggling with sleep. My brother would let me listen to his transistor radio to help me fall asleep. The radio had a leather cover. Today, the smell of leather can bring back that memory of lying in bed and waiting for sleep to come. While nothing was verbalized, I was aware of the love and compassion of our church and community.

We were changed by the grief we carried. Life was no longer lighthearted. Our mother had to gain full-time employment. She was fortunate enough to get a job at the local post office. It was a godsend. Jobs in our small town were at a premium, especially ones with benefits. The hours allowed her to still be available to her elderly parents and her young family.

Since Mom was the newest employee, she worked seven days a week. She reported directly to the post office on Monday through Saturday. On Sundays, she would meet the early-morning mail train and take the mail back to the post office. Before sorting the mail, she would go next door to the town laundromat and fill up a row of washers with our dirty laundry. Returning to the post office, she sorted the mail while the clothes washed. Completing her work, she would lock the post office, dry the clothes, and return home with our clean laundry for the week—just in time for lunch.

Because our mother was so busy, Marylee and I helped with the cooking and household chores. Looking back, I can laugh at some of our early attempts at unsupervised cooking and baking. I remember the time I added extra food coloring to my potato salad. It turned out orange, but we still ate it. I recall baking a cake and hiding it under the bed to surprise her when she came home from work later that night. I always wondered how she felt about the cake that had been sitting under the dusty bed. Marylee, who liked to iron, would help with that chore. This was before perma-press was invented, so it was an arduous task.

Rodney, the oldest and only boy, felt the loss deeply. He had spent a lot of time with our father. Rodney tells the story of riding with Daddy to Galesburg, thirty miles away, to get a load of gravel for the roads. He felt important and grown-up when he was with Daddy. With our father's death, he was the only male in the household. Rodney had dyslexia issues like our father. He remembers how our father struggled with reading and math. He lost the only parent who understood his challenges. The three of us worked together to survive our trauma and support our mother. Now, many years later, we remain close and supportive of one another.

Even with our father's death, our childhood was never depicted as sad. Marylee and I did not think of it that way. Grief and the loss of our father were not discussed. I only saw my mother cry once. I do not recall my mother complaining about her responsibilities as she became the sole breadwinner and only parent. Our family did not focus on the difficulties; we were taught to go forward, to do our best, and to find the happy. It was the best lesson of our childhood and has carried all of us far.

CHAPTER 2

The Teen Years

Young love, first love, filled with true devotion,
Young love, our love, share with deep emotion.
—Ric Cartey

On my sixteenth birthday, I met the man I would marry. Boyd Christy, a recent transplant to Illinois, met my cousin. The two guys became friends. Upon meeting Boyd, Aunt Franny immediately took Boyd under her wing. She soon became a second mother to him. When she heard the boys discussing looking for girls to date, Aunt Franny suggested introducing Boyd to me.

As I write this fifty years later, it is astonishing to me that this really happened. We were both so young! In truth, I was probably more mature than most sixteen-year-olds, having responsibilities due to my father's death four years earlier. Boyd was mature because his parents were divorced. He felt responsible for his younger brother.

Boyd and I dated throughout high school, two starry-eyed teenagers. Not living in the same town, we didn't see each other during the week and counted the days until the weekends. Boyd played on the basketball team. I can see in my mind's eye the handsome guy with a crew cut running out onto the basketball court. I was in the band at my high school. Boyd would come to the football games while I marched. A magical night for us was the prom. I had a beautiful pink gown with a hoop skirt, and Boyd's cousin loaned him his red Falcon convertible to drive. We were young and in love.

Boyd and I were destined to be married, yet I felt pulled to fulfill a life of faith-based service. When I was seventeen, my church sponsored an opportunity to attend a weeklong tour of the Methodist missions throughout Illinois. This experience fanned the fire of service to others I had already felt and opened my eyes to opportunities in the realm of Christian service. I was exposed to multiple missions as we traveled around the state, and I felt a growing desire to have a career that helped others. Most memorable were Hull House in Chicago and the Baby Fold in Normal. Both were ministries to help children and families in need. I can still picture the babies in the Baby Fold nursery waiting to be adopted. I found it easy to envision myself participating in that type of career. Along with exposing me to many possibilities for service, this experience validated my gifts of leadership. In my own family, I was teased for being a "bossy-cat." I realized that leadership ability was a gift. I began to feel confident in allowing those gifts to blossom.

By my senior year in high school, I felt pressure to decide what career direction I would take upon graduation. In the early sixties in a small town, combining career and family was not seen as the norm. Girls did one of four things: nurse, teacher, secretary, or wife/ mother. I was smart and had some counselors pushing me to go to college. My mother was a widow and had no idea about sending me to college. I was in love and wanted to get married and consummate that love. I had watched my mother raise three children alone, and I was motivated to develop a marketable skill.

As I considered different career possibilities, nursing was appealing. I felt it would be a good choice. Nursing could be a vocation I would be able to merge with my desire to be a mother and wife, fulfilling my desire to serve others. However, my dream of attending nursing school after high school became complicated. In the 1960s, nursing students were not allowed to be married, and cohabitation was not accepted in our culture. I found a licensed practical nurse program that was one year long and located within commuting distance, which enabled me to live at home. My mother could afford the tuition. I enrolled, purchased a car, and was ready to go.

When I started nursing school, my horizons began to broaden. I made the daily commute into a larger city and found myself challenged with a whole new environment. Wearing my white oxfords, white stockings, and the required green pinafore and a white blouse, I started my schooling, which would lead me to a vocation I would enjoy for many years.

The first six months were academic and included the study of biology, anatomy and physiology, pharmacology, nutrition, and nursing practices. The second half of the year included patient care in the hospital, and I was exposed to myriad people and situations. Hands-on nursing experiences included providing bed baths, feeding patients, emptying bedpans, and giving nightly back rubs, as well as medications, injections, and other skills. Serving in this way was not always easy for a small-town girl, but gaining skills for comforting others felt good.

While I was busy studying nursing, Marylee was enjoying her last two years of high school. With her extroverted personality, she became involved in all kinds of activities, including being a cheerleader. Her favorite subjects were secretarial courses and home economics. During high school, she dated Bob Ulm, a young man who she cared for deeply. Bob was three years older than Marylee. He worked in a factory along with his father and brothers.

Marylee's love affair wasn't just with Bob—but with the whole close-knit family. Bob's parents, Ruth and Laurance Ulm, were happily married and opened their hearts to Marylee, filling the gaping hole in her heart left by the death of our father.

She writes:

> Besides my own parents, I suspect that these
> two had the most impact on my life and helped

shape me in many ways. The first time I met Ruth and Laurance, I was instantly drawn to them. I loved how they cared for each other, how they teased each other, and saw their deep love for their marriage and family.

Ruth and Laurance seemed to enjoy having me around, and before long, I was a part of the family gatherings on Sunday nights. The whole family would get together for food, conversation, and fun. Sometimes the fun was just a conversation or discussion, but many times, especially in the later years, there were games, old movies, looking at photo albums, and digging through the cedar chest (where Ruth kept the "good" nightgowns in case she ever went to the hospital). I was always drawn to their affection for each other, openly touching and exchanging smiles. For an impressionable young woman, this was heaven.

In October 1965, I graduated from nursing school, and eight days later, Boyd and I were married in a small wedding. I began my nursing career at a local hospital. We found a duplex to rent within walking distance of the hospital. Boyd was in school and worked part-time. We were happy to be together and ready to build our life.

Marylee graduated from high school the following May. Marylee and Bob married in September 1966 and set up housekeeping in an apartment in Farmington. Marylee looked for some type of secretarial work, but with Bob working full-time, there was no pressure to find employment.

Marylee and I were two happy young brides, confident in our futures. We were also naïve with a very limited views of the world. As we began our lives, our perception of what those lives would be was narrow. We envisioned happy marriages, wonderful children, and simple lives in Farmington. We had little understanding of the wider world, but God had much bigger lives for us than we could envision.

CHAPTER 3

Boyd Dale Christy

Death leaves a heartache no one can heal,
Love leaves a memory no one can steal.
—Author unknown

Eight days before our first anniversary, and two weeks after Marylee's wedding, our first son was born. We named him Boyd Dale Christy. Even though we were not financially ready, the baby was welcomed with great joy and happiness. I was amazed and surprised at my intense love for him.

Boyd and I were both twenty years old and felt fortunate to have our little baby boy. We were optimistic and very much in love. Neither of us felt like we were missing out on a social life or freedom. Our little family was our joy and happiness. Financially, we were living paycheck to paycheck. When Boyd Dale was three months old, we decided I needed to return to work. Boyd worked the day shift, and I found a job on the second shift. Boyd Dale would be with one of his parents the majority of the time.

Boyd was very involved in our son's care. He would be insulted if someone suggested he was babysitting. He was Boyd Dale's father, an equal parent, and we worked as a team. I would put a load of clothes in the washer before going to work, and he would hang them up on hangers and a rack to dry during the night since we didn't have a dryer. I would arrive home from work and find my little family

15

sleeping. While this meant Boyd and I had less time together, we were satisfied with our life. We were young and strong and ready to work hard. Since I was home during the day, I loved to take Boyd Dale over to visit my grandparents. Housebound, my elderly grandparents were pleased when I would drop in to tell them about my life. I was thrilled to share my sweet baby with them. I would set him on each of their laps. My grandfather, who had limited eyesight, would move his head to try to see Boyd Dale's face. My grandmother would tell me how strong he was and share her wisdom of child-rearing.

Marylee said, "I was enchanted with becoming an aunt and hugely romanticized my sister's life with a handsome husband and a beautiful baby."

In those early months, Marylee and I would get together for lunch. Bob, Marylee, Boyd, and I, with Boyd Dale in tow, would get together with other young married couples in our small town to socialize.

Our joyful life, however, was short-lived. On a cold February night, I arrived home from work at midnight and found our four-month-old son dead in his crib, a victim of SIDS (sudden infant death syndrome). There are no words to describe the pain and shock of that event, and we did not possess the courage to look at it closely. We numbly went through the rituals that surround death. We borrowed money from my brother to buy a burial plot and had a graveside service for our beloved son.

I shall not forget the coldness of that February morn: walking across the frozen earth to that little blue coffin and facing the horror that this was happening to me. My baby was gone. We were not encouraged to openly grieve, but family surrounded us with love and support. While Boyd and I were at my mother's, my aunt went into our home and removed the baby's crib and all his clothes. This was the family's well-intentioned way of protecting us from further suffering. Boyd found a bib, which comforted him, and carried it in his pocket for a long time. I did not see any of the baby things until we were preparing for our daughter's birth five years later. When I did go through his things, I felt happy to finally be using them again. We used the crib that we had excitedly purchased for our firstborn for all of our five babies.

With Boyd Dale's death, Marylee's life changed as well. Our mother arrived at Marylee's apartment to tell her of his death. The news was devastating. The fantasy that she and I so strongly believed in had been destroyed. Marylee remembered thinking how unfair this all was and that no one could possibly recover from such a loss. The days surrounding his death were a blur, and she felt totally helpless—as we all did. Again, two sisters were grieving together.

In deep grief, having a supportive listening ear is a precious gift. Marylee provided her support then, and we have been that for each other for our whole lives.

I realized that I would never again experience unqualified joy. I lost a sense of innocence and purity. No matter what other wonderful things came into my life, I would carry the grief. However, I did not want the pain to dominate my life. I wanted to believe that good things would come. I needed to embrace the belief that bad things happen to everyone—and mine came early.

CHAPTER 4

The Vietnam War

Still I Rise.
—Maya Angelou

In the midst of our family pain, the rest of the world was being ravaged by the Vietnam War. The second shock came when a short six weeks after Boyd Dale's death, Boyd received his draft notice. Although my husband initially had been spared from the draft due to Boyd Dale's birth, his name was now moved to the top of the list, and he was drafted into the US Army. It was a direct path to serving in the infantry in Vietnam. In October 1967, he got on a plane bound for Vietnam.

I took Boyd to the airport. As I watched his plane leave, I wondered what the future held. *Would he survive—or would he die?* I remained in Illinois, working, taking college classes, and waiting for his return, hoping we would be able to rebuild our lives. While he was gone, Marylee and I continued to socialize and be intimately involved in each other's lives. We would get together to cook and were quite proud when we mastered tacos, which seemed like an exotic dish to us.

I had not thought about the possibility of Boyd being seriously injured. On January 15, 1968, Boyd was gravely wounded. I did not have to endure the frightening experience of having army personnel come to the door to tell me my husband was seriously wounded, which was the policy at the time. Instead, I learned of his injury through a letter that a Red Cross volunteer had written.

On a cold Sunday morning in January, I went to the post office to check my mail. I found an envelope with Red Cross lettering and unfamiliar red handwriting. What a frightening moment! The letter had been dictated by Boyd to a Red Cross worker. Boyd didn't realize it at the time, but it had been three days since the injury. He had been unconscious, undergoing several surgeries during that time. I received little specific information about his injury. He did say his leg was broken. Not realizing the seriousness of his injuries, I was thankful. I reasoned that they wouldn't keep him in-country to wait on a bone to heal. He would be coming home alive.

Boyd recalled that the company was ambushed, he was shot in the right leg, a medic tied a rag around his leg, and he was transferred by a vehicle and then in a helicopter to an inflatable MASH (military army surgical hospital) unit. He said, "I remember waking up and the guy next to me said, 'We're going to make it because this isn't where they put the soldiers who are dying.'" He has no recollection of exactly how many surgeries he had in Vietnam and then in Japan. The main artery of his right leg had been severed. They transplanted a vein from the left leg to function as an artery in the right. It was an experimental treatment at the time, and many years later, a vascular surgeon was amazed that he still had blood flow to that foot. The leg was saved, but due to the blood loss, he developed gangrene. Much of the tissue and bone had to be removed. Boyd has lived with the possibility of amputation for much of his life.

Near the one-year anniversary of our son's death, I got the call. Boyd had just landed in California and would be going to Fitzsimmons Army Hospital in Denver, Colorado. I was at work when I got the call. I remember running down the halls, so excited and thankful. He was coming home, and I was going to Denver!

We were fortunate. My aunt and uncle lived close to Fitzsimmons, and they were a great support. I found an apartment, applied for a nursing license in Colorado, and found a job. Our joy of being reunited overshadowed the difficult parts of his rehabilitation and trauma. We thrived.

A military hospital at the height of the Vietnam War was nothing like the hospitals of today. The wards were full of wounded men: long rows with curtains between probably forty or more in a ward. There were no televisions or other types of entertainment in the wards. Reading books and playing cards or games filled the time. Our favorite game was cribbage. We played more than two hundred games, keeping tally of who was ahead in the competition. Fitzsimmons was a small army complex that included a theater with an area to accommodate stretchers and wheelchairs. I would push his wheelchair over to the theater and bring a stool to prop up his leg while we enjoyed a movie.

During the year of his treatment, there were periods when Boyd would be able to live at the apartment and go to the hospital for different types of outpatient treatments. Then he would be admitted for a surgery, eventually returning to outpatient status. Living in a large metropolitan city was a new experience, and we found lots of advantages: large supermarkets, a mall, diversity, and restaurants. Often Boyd would be in a cast and on crutches, but we could still go play mini-golf or take car trips up into the mountains, often inviting wounded friends to join us. The mountain trips were very healing, and I would feel the presence of God in his majestic mountains. All of a sudden, we saw a much wider world than the small-town life we had experienced. Our time in Colorado was filled many happy memories. We were very thankful for his survival and enjoyed life together.

While Boyd and I were living in Denver, Marylee and Bob purchased a house in Middlegrove, Illinois, population one hundred, a few miles west of Farmington. All of Bob's family lived there, and Marylee enjoyed being part of the clan. Marylee was happy creating their first home.

While Marylee and I were living a thousand miles apart, we wrote letters and occasionally talked on the phone. Marylee recalled that it was important knowing that Boyd was safe and that we would eventually be able to return home. Marylee and Bob came to Colorado to visit us, and Marylee found the reunion healing. We spent time in the mountains and enjoyed tourist activities while they visited. We could see our life was going to return to normal.

After fifteen months of treatment, Boyd retired from the army. He was ready to return to civilian life. His right leg had been classified as 100 percent disabled, which meant the function was equal to a below-the-knee amputation. He was fitted with a brace and a built-up shoe. While our Colorado friends teased that we would return to the mountains, we were ready go home where our family and friends lived. Boyd returned to Caterpillar, Inc. and was assigned a desk job due to his disability. He enjoyed a thirty-eight-year career in the benefits department before he retired. I found a job working for a pediatrician. Normalcy returned.

In September 1969, Marylee gave birth to their first son, Kent. Marylee felt complete. Her dream of becoming a wife and mother had come true. She was content. Marylee was able to secure a little part-time job sorting the mail each day for the hundred or so residents of Middlegrove. The postal station was in the corner of the little gas station/restaurant that her in-laws ran. As an extrovert, she enjoyed interacting with people and loved bringing her little guy along with her to sort the mail every morning. This continued until after her second son, Matthew, was born and her mother-in-law took over the mail sorting.

In April 1970, our daughter, Molly Frances, was born, and we bought our first home. As wonderful as these blessings were, I felt unsettled. I had experienced all these difficult, mind-expanding experiences, and I was struggling with the normalcy of being a stay-at-home mom with housework as my daily focus.

God was preparing us for something bigger. A yearning was growing in me. I saw the return to Illinois as a time when I was going to pick up the threads of my old life, but I couldn't because I was not the same person as when I left. Both Boyd and I had changed and grown and learned some important life lessons.

CHAPTER 5

Our Adoption Story

*We are mosaics—pieces of light, love, history, stars—
glued together with magic and music and words.*
—Anita Krishan

A voracious reader, I would fill my mind and days with reading while Molly napped. I read a book about a family who had adopted multiple children with special needs and different ethnicities. The author's description of the story she used to explain her children differences in skin color inspired me. Simple and beautiful, she told them that when God was creating each child, they ended up in the oven at different times, thus the different shades. I loved the thought of a house full of children and the richness of multiple skin shades, each contributing to the family. I pictured a great adventure. Boyd and I longed for more children, and even though I knew we could have more biological children, I felt unsettled. My heart knew that biology wasn't as important as love, and I had an innate knowledge God was preparing a ministry for us. I believed God placed this discontent within my heart to awaken the thought of adopting a child who needed a home. I needed to see if Boyd felt the same way.

When I shared this desire with him, he admitted it wasn't something he had ever considered, but he listened. However, as he was driving home one day, he heard God's voice, which convinced him that adoption was our family's calling. Little did we know the unbelievable journey our lives would take as we pursued enlarging our family through adoption.

We contacted an agency and inquired about adoption. We were invited to come to an informational meeting for the possible placement of what in 1970s terms was called a "hard-to-place" child. While we did not have a specific plan for exactly what this type of adoption might entail, we were confident that adoption was right for us. At the meeting, we heard about different types of children, their challenges, and the adoption process. As we listened to the stories of several white couples who had adopted black children, we felt that this was a match for us. The warning of the possibility of losing relationships with our families and friends and being treated with prejudice did not deter our desire to adopt across racial lines. We thought it sounded exciting and fulfilling. Our belief was undergirded through our faith. We had found our calling!

In 1971, however, a movement developed by the National Association of Black Social Workers who believed that too many white couples were adopting black children without addressing the racial needs of the child. We were met with concern and possible hostility from many in this community. All of a sudden, the tables turned. We would be "stealing their children." How could a white couple teach a child to cope with racial slurs and unfair treatment if they themselves had no idea what that was like? What about appreciating and valuing their African American roots? What about their ability to function comfortably within the local black community? What about skin and hair care? What about friends? In our case, there would also be the issue of a black child growing up in a small town where a child could be treated as the "token" black. Eventually, the child would be faced with the challenge of leaving our small town and be unprepared to live in the larger world of racism.

The agency we were working with made it clear to us that we would have to educate and dedicate ourselves to meeting these concerns. We attended a conference in Saint Louis and prepared ourselves. We learned about the possible backlash of responses for bringing a black child into our home. Questions arose like, "What will you do if your extended family rejects you?" We learned about developing a lifestyle that would include diversity as well as seeing that our adopted child would have significant black adults in his/her life so that he/she would be prepared to function well in society as an adult. The lessons we were presented were very clear. We would be forever changed. We embraced the challenge. Ultimately, the agency approved us, and we excitedly waited for a child. Our wait felt very different than the preparation for a biological birth. We didn't have a due date or even a known age of the child we would be receiving. We had agreed to a placement of any child under the age of two, preferring a boy.

We began to prepare for this big change in our life. In addition to the usual second child adjustments, we would be adjusting to new challenges of parenting a brown-skinned child. Our family would no longer be Caucasian; we would be multicultural. We shared our plans with family and friends. We knew creating an "integrated" toy box was important in normalizing and embracing diversity.

The following Christmas I searched diligently for a black baby doll for Molly. I searched for books with children of color. The first I found was *The Snowy Day* by Ezra Jack Keats, published in 1962, one of the first popular children's books with a brown-skinned child. A few years later, Molly asked for a popular anatomically correct boy doll for Christmas: a black version, like her brother. I could not find one in the farming area where we lived, but a friend purchased the doll in Chicago and mailed it to me. We subscribed to *Ebony* magazine and were interested in black issues of the time. As the children matured, we celebrated Martin Luther King Jr. Day with an activity that enhanced our children's racial identities. One year, our family went to hear Nelson Mandela's daughter speak at a Chicago church as part of the Martin Luther King holiday weekend.

In April 1972, we got the call from the agency offering the placement of a month-old biracial (black/white) baby boy. It was an exciting day of joy for our little family of three. The agency orchestrated the adoption day, and we reported to the foster home to see "the baby." Upon meeting him, we were ready to seal the deal and take him home. However, the social worker insisted on taking us out for lunch so we could discuss the adoption of this specific child. We were confident that we were capable of handling this biracial placement. I had been forewarned by other adoptive parents that the agency could stop the proceedings, and that terrified me. They held all the cards. We wanted this baby, and they had the power. I also believe that the agency was very nervous about doing their first placement of black child in a white home.

I wanted to prove that I was the perfect mom, and when we went out to lunch with the social worker, I was very nervous. I had succumbed the belief of the era: good mothers had their children potty-trained at age two. Molly was two and was in the middle of that process. Before the invention of disposable diapers, I had her in heavy training pants, praying that we wouldn't have any "accidents."

Just as we were sitting down, Molly announced she needed to go "potty."

I hopped up and headed for the restroom with her. It was a long distance from where we were sitting. When we arrived, I discovered pay toilets, and I had no coins to unlock a stall. I panicked! Can she hold it long enough for us to run back to the table to get my purse? What will the social worker think? Rather than facing these fears, I got down on my hands and knees and crawled under the stall to open the door for Molly. Her pants were still dry! We arrived back at the lunch table unscathed. After lunch and paperwork, we returned to the foster home and claimed our newest family member: a beautiful baby boy. We named him Rod William.

Rod's arrival home was the talk of the town. People had a difficult time understanding our motivation. In their minds, having biological children was best, so why would we bring a "stranger" into our family? The racial issues added even more confusion for them. Without even realizing it, these well-intentioned white people were racist, however subtle and unaware, and this child made them uncomfortable. Some form of racism is ingrained in all of us, and they were unaware that they held those feelings until confronted with his brown face and kinky hair. In contrast, we saw our son as a beautiful gift from God and delighted in his brown skin, tight hair, and other cultural customs. Life was exciting as we learned proper care of his hair.

The first months after the adoption, we were treated very well. Initially, our life didn't change significantly. Friends held a surprise baby shower for us and made an attempt to show their support. I had an encounter with the local priest. In an attempt to complement our decision, he said it was better to adopt a child needing a home than to adopt a dog. As time went on, social invitations became less frequent. Community members found it difficult to adjust to the changes they saw in our family. We had been trained to be very vigilant against racial prejudice. As our son grew, race became a divisive barrier that couldn't be overcome.

Within our own family, one set of grandparents wanted to claim our biological daughter Molly as their granddaughter, but they would ignore Rod as a grandchild. We chose to limit their contact. Our family was all four of us—or no one. Others embraced his arrival and loved him as they loved Molly. My mother had a sister who asked that he not be mentioned in any of her letters, but the rest of her family had no issues. My father's family also accepted him with no reservations.

As part of the adoption process, we were introduced to a chapter of the North American Council on Adoptable Children (NACAC) and were encouraged to attend monthly meetings where we could network with other families who had also adopted across racial lines. With the mission statement of "because every child deserves a permanent, loving, and culturally competent family," this local group was our support. We made lifelong friends for ourselves and for our children, and our life expanded in many ways. Our children grew up knowing white families, black families, and mixed-up families like ours. We had farmer friends and Chicago friends, church friends, school friends, neighborhood friends … we enjoyed a wonderful richness of people as our family grew, each in his own uniqueness.

When Rod was turning two, we realized we were ready to relocate to an integrated environment. We needed to live where there were other brown-skinned kids in the neighborhood and schools. Boyd and I wanted to build more relationships with a more diverse population. We sold our home and moved our family to Peoria, Illinois. We settled into our new home, ready to embrace a new lifestyle. We had found our calling. We had two delightful kids with every intention of adding to our family.

CHAPTER 6

A Growing Family

Nothing can dim the light that shines from within.
—Maya Angelou

At that point in my life, I thought I had accomplished much and was anticipating our life with a happy family, adopting more children, providing them a good life, educating them, teaching them to cope with the ups and downs of life, and sending them out into the world. God's hand is omnipotent, and we were heading into a new and painful challenge.

The bottom fell out of my life plan when Rod was diagnosed with cystic fibrosis, an incurable genetic disease. When Boyd Dale died, I remember thinking, *I got through that because it was over suddenly. I could never stand knowing my child had an incurable disease.* I was now facing that scenario. Learning your child is not expected to live into adulthood is devastating and challenging. I struggled with sleep, cried many private tears, and often felt overwhelmed. More importantly, I had two lively, adorable children who needed a happy involved mom. Our deep faith with the love and determination we felt in our calling to parent these children, propelled Boyd and me forward to embrace each day.

Rod's illness required daily medical care, which included physical therapy, aerosol treatments, and medications. Rod would inhale a medicated aerosol to thin the sticky mucus in his lungs, and then Boyd or I would administer the therapy by thumping on his chest, focusing on specific positions. This process would help him expectorate the mucus that plugged his lungs and compromised his breathing. We performed this treatment twice a day when he was healthy and four times a day when he was sick. Rod was not always cooperative, but I had a jar of pennies, and when he laid still and coughed, he got a penny. We would stack them up as we worked our way through his therapy.

Although Rod was chronically ill, we enjoyed the normal activities of a young family: trips to the park, bike rides, picnics, ball games, and family vacations. In some ways, our life was further enriched as we learned to live one day at a time. Rod had an outgoing, feisty personality. There was no slowing down and feeling sorry for yourself. God had prepared Rod to live his life to the fullest—even if it was going to be short. We embraced a philosophy that life was to be lived, and so we did.

Three years later, having adjusted to life that included Rod's medical needs, we were ready to expand our family. We decided there should be two brown faces at the table rather than one, and we started the process of adopting another biracial baby. We, once again, experienced the ups and downs of the adoption process: a social worker was in the driver's seat concerning the approval and placement of another child.

After a relatively uneventful home study, we were offered a baby girl with a cleft lip and palate and big beautiful brown eyes. I put her picture on the refrigerator, ready for the call to complete her placement. She had a final court date, and she would be ours. The judge decided to delay release of parental rights, and we had to wait another month before she could be placed. For me, it was a long month of looking at her picture. I wanted to hold her in my arms. Finally, on March 25, 1976, our family of four went to the adoption agency excited to bring our baby girl home. Molly, a kindergartener, announced it was "B-day" because we were getting a baby. Rod, at four, was always ready for an adventure and happily joined along in the family event.

At the agency, we were taken to a small room to spend time with our new baby, who we named Melissa Ann. Six-month-old Melissa was very frightened meeting this roomful of strangers, and she cried inconsolably. After what seemed like an eternity, we were allowed to change her into the clothes we brought and take her home. I recall thinking, *there is a foster mom somewhere crying also.* Melissa's crying continued until a nap in the afternoon. She awoke bright-eyed and happy. Except for adolescence, she has stayed that way.

Becoming a member of our family was an adjustment for Melissa. She had been in the care of her birth mother and then a foster mother before her placement. She was wary of women, and once she was bonded to me, all other women were a threat. However, she was always happy to have a man pick her up. Rodney would tease my mother that Melissa liked him better.

A few months after Melissa's placement, my dear friend Ellen, who loved caring for babies, kept her for the day. Ellen was disappointed because had to leave Melissa in the playpen for much of the day. Every time Ellen picked up Melissa, she cried. Selfishly, as an experienced mother, the biggest thrill for me was her habit of sleeping twelve hours every night. From the first night in our home, she would cocoon herself in the blankets and go off to sleep. After she was asleep, I would quietly sneak in and uncover her head.

The addition of a child with cleft lip and palate might sound daunting, but for our family, it seemed right. We had good health insurance, and with my background in nursing, the prospect of multiple surgeries and ongoing care was not intimidating. Our family already had a dad with a physical handicap that required continued medical attention and a son with a respiratory disease, so the addition of a child with a cleft lip and palate was hardly noticed. We lived with a positive attitude. In our family, it was normal to ask, "Who needs to go to the hospital next?"

Looking back, I recognize that God was continuing to mold my life in amazing ways I couldn't see. I must admit the spring I had Boyd and Rod at home receiving intravenous antibiotics at the same time was overwhelming. Neither Rod nor Melissa nor Boyd stood out since they all had their different medical needs. Those needs were treated as simply a part of life. Life was full and busy—a very happy period for us.

CHAPTER 7

Rod William Christy

No one is you, and that is your power.
—Emily Manassah

Rod was unique in personality and spirit. I thought I understood God's purposes in giving us Rod, but Rod's purposes were higher than I could understand. In his short life, he inspired many to keep going. It is my delight to write about him. The great love I have for him, along with his siblings, is a joy to share. He has been in heaven for many years, and his friends, cousins, and siblings have all grown into adults with families of their own. However, I would guess everyone who remembers him has a story about him. Rod was always intent on being noticed. He often operated with the belief that negative attention was better than no attention. Rod suffered from an incurable disease that left him small and thin with a chronic cough, yet he was not remembered for his illness. He was remembered for his energy and vibrant personality. Six months after his death, the elementary school Rod had attended planted a tree in his memory. All his classmates wrote "Remembering Rod" cards. Not one card mentioned his illness, but they all mentioned a classmate who had them all convinced that his "brown muscles" were stronger and faster.

His sisters were very aware of his illness, and they lived with the daily therapy, pills, and hospitalizations. We tried to keep his care part of our normal family culture. As with all siblings, they had the usual ups and downs. Each of his sisters has stories of his antics. One of Rod's main aggravations for his older sister, Molly, occurred as they walked to school in the mornings. He would slowly tap his toes as they walked, slowing down the trip and making her nervous that they might be late. Even more irritating, per Molly, was his habit of saving extra gum and uneaten candy in his room. Melissa, his younger sister, identified closely to her brother. They were both adopted and were the two brown faces at the dinner table. Rod loved sports, and so did Melissa. Rod's best friend, John, and his younger brother, Billy, lived across the street. The four kids were always playing a game: baseball in the spring and summer, football and basketball in the fall and winter. Only during Rod's last year of life did his health affect his ability to participate in sports. However, he was included as part of the group, finding a less strenuous role.

Rod was blessed with two male cousins, Marylee's sons, Matt and Kent. These cousins lived in our hometown of Farmington, twenty-five miles from where we lived in Peoria. Marylee shares her recollections of the first time Rod spent the night with his cousins. In her words, she shares the story of one simple weekend when a beautiful little brown boy got to have a sleepover with his two white blond cousins. Matthew, Marylee's younger son, was the same age as Rod. Kent, her firstborn, was two years older.

I had looked forward to this weekend for several reasons. While my sons had gotten to know their cousin through family gatherings, it always felt like the time was cut short and didn't allow much "little boy" playing time. I think my boys secretly felt because Rod had sisters, he missed the benefit of a brother. I remember whenever we were together, the three of them always enjoyed playing together.

Because Rod had cystic fibrosis, he needed therapy twice daily. He hadn't been able to be away from home since his parents were the primary caregivers who were skilled in doing his therapy. They taught me to how to do his therapy. While I felt was competent doing it, I was still a bit nervous wanting to do everything perfect.

The time finally arrived when Rod came to our house for an overnight. My boys were thrilled to have him visit. Those who knew Rod wouldn't be surprised that even though he was only about four or five, he tried to negotiate not having his evening treatment. I was adamant that everything would be done to perfection. Bath time was approaching, and I said that the three of them could take a bath together, but therapy was first. The excitement of hopping in the tub with his cousins and their toys was carrot enough for Rod to agree to participate actively in his therapy. My boys watched with interest as we proceeded. First was breathing the medicated mist and then his laying in several positions as I pounded with cupped hands the different lobes of his lungs and encouraged coughing and spitting the thick gunk from his lungs. I remember feeling quite triumphant following that first treatment I did on my own.

Next, I drew the bathwater, added bubbles, and tossed in three little boys and their toys. I watched for a while, then stepped away from for a little bit to let them laugh, play, and be boys. I remember looking at that dark-skinned boy next to my two blonds and thought, *outside, they are so different, but that's where it ends. Inside, they are just the same.* I can still remember looking at Rod's wiry, skinny body, noticing his thin legs and bottom, but sporting that barrel chest, a typical body shape for kids with cystic fibrosis. I was fully aware he would likely not live to adulthood, but I distinctly remember thinking in that moment that he'd probably live to be twenty or so, thinking that wouldn't be so bad. It's interesting how our minds play games with reality. No matter when we would lose him, it would be horrible. I also remember thinking that if he died and my son, who was the same age lived on, how my sister could ever stand to be around us. I imagined the pain would be too much for her to endure. But this evening was all about the fun of boys being boys. I stuffed those feelings somewhere deep and moved on as that "special" aunt who had two sons.

When it was time to get out and put on pajamas, I lathered my boys' hair as usual and then moved on to Rod's kinky black crown. I discovered his hair was quite different than my blond-headed boys. What I thought was short, once washed, was much longer. Once Rod was dried and in pajamas, it was time for me to comb his hair. I did not have the right equipment or products. I remember we ended up with a dry, knotted, and rather wild "fro." I learned later that his type of hair didn't get washed daily and needed oils and products to keep it soft. I happily learned before the next sleepover the proper hair care for that little guy: using a pick and some Afro-Sheen. This was the first of several sleepovers we had over the next few years, and each one was meaningful for me and barrels of fun for the boys.

Kent shares a story of Rod's impact on a young man named Bruce who lived down the street from Kent. The young man, who was biracial, had recently moved to Farmington and was struggling with being accepted because of his race. A child navigating racism in a small town is challenging. He discovered that Kent and Matt's cousin, Rod, was biracial and was loved and accepted by them. From that day forward, he knew that he would be welcomed into their home as well. Matt and Kent's sensitivity was heightened to racial inequalities by living in Rod's world, and so were the lives of many others.

Several times a year, Rod would be hospitalized with pneumonia, which required a two-week stay. Required to be isolated in his room, fourteen days was a long time for a little boy to be content with his mom, a television, and some card games. He got busy devising creative ways to engage additional people. One day, the hospital's activity therapist set up an air hockey game in his room. Besides the fun of playing the game, he would be delighted when curious people would wander in to see which happy child was making all the noise.

During one of his hospitalizations, Rod needed wall suction and had to be in a private room on an adult floor. Once again, he was looking for action. He had a remote-control car that he would drive into the hall in hopes of gaining attention. One day, a little nun came into his room to investigate who was driving the car. How his eyes danced when he was successful in connecting with another person.

Learning to swallow air so he could burp loudly was yet another way to attract somebody's attention from the hospital halls. He loved to engage others in his antics. As scary and heart-wrenching as it was dealing with his disease, he kept us in the present with his personality, love of people, and passion for life. He lived a life filled with fight and taught us to engage in our world each and every day.

Boyd loved basketball. He had played in high school. When we moved within walking distance of Bradley University, Boyd became an avid fan and shared his love with Rod. From the time Rod could walk, his favorite toy was a ball. I fixed many meals while he shot at a hoop attached to the kitchen door. Rod and his dad attended many games in 1976, when he was four. The next year Boyd, Rod, and his uncle Rodney—who he was named for—purchased season tickets. Rod had an unusual understanding of the sport. The three guys rarely missed a game. Once when Rod was very sick and a patient in adult ICU, he talked the nurses into finding a portable television so he could watch a Bradley game.

Bradley's home games were played in the Robertson Memorial Fieldhouse on the university campus. The building was two converted B-29 airplane hangars from WWII combined. The arena was unique because the floor was raised, and with the red-painted apron, it gave the appearance of a stage. The roof was curved, and the eight thousand fans sat in stacked seating. The closeness of the fans and the reverberating noise from the ceiling gave the Braves a home-court advantage.

Rod, his dad, and his uncle developed a routine for all the home games. Arriving early, they would enter the fieldhouse and go stand in the hall outside the locker room. That spot gave Rod the opportunity to have the players hit his hand as they ran out. Next, they would move to the edge of the raised floor. Rod would have his dad lift him up on the floor as they watched the warm-ups. When the players headed back to locker room, Boyd, Rod, and Rodney would head up into the bleachers to watch the game. At halftime, they purchased a snack of popcorn and soda pop. Rod insisted on staying until the game was over—regardless if either team was ahead by a large margin. He would repeat the score out loud to remember. When they returned home, he would walk into the house and announce the final score.

Cousin Matt shared his memories when he came from Farmington to attend a Bradley Basketball game with his cousin and uncles. He, too, followed their routine. He remembers the fieldhouse, which was very large with large crowds. The four guys held hands as they snaked their way through the throng and climbed the wooden stairs up to their seats. Matt remembers a Bradley game after Rod's death where he was the honorary ball boy. He sat on the sidelines, knowing his cousin's spirit was right beside him.

In 1980, Bradley won the Missouri Valley Conference championship and a trip to the NCAA Tournament. The team would be playing in Denton, Texas. The Bradley Brave Booster Club organized a plane trip to the game, and Boyd and I discussed the possibility of taking Rod on the trip. Rod's health was stable, but we knew it was unlikely he would survive to adulthood. We decided the trip would be a wonderful experience for them to share. Rod's first and only plane ride and being taken out of school added to the excitement.

Boyd loved taking his gregarious, outgoing son. With Rod's sparkling and charming personality, he could be quite the young chick magnet. While in Denton, they went to a postgame team party, and Boyd got separated from Rod. He found Rod sitting on the piano bench next to a pretty cheerleader. Two years later, when Rod died, we were very thankful we made the choice we did.

CHAPTER 8

Family Camp

In happy moments, praise God.
In difficult moments, seek God.
In quiet moments, trust God.
In every moment, thank God.
—Rick Warren

Early in Rod's life, God began laying the first stepping-stone to create a life and ministry much greater than our adoption story. A simple decision of our young family attending a family church camp led to the current ministry of stroke camp weekends. Today, hundreds of stroke survivors and caregivers enjoy a renewing weekend retreat birthed from our early experiences at a camp.

In the summer of 1972, my mother stopped by our home with a church brochure for a weeklong family church camp at a nearby Methodist campground. She thought it sounded like a fun getaway and suggested that our family join her and my brother, Rodney, in attending. Sounding like a nice low-cost getaway for our young family, we decided to attend. We would enjoy a break in our routine, and I wouldn't have to cook or do dishes for a week. No cooking and no dishes cinched it for me, and the six of us registered.

We were familiar with the beautiful eighty-acre haven. Epworth Springs Camp was owned and operated by the United Methodist Church. Located in the rolling farmland of central Illinois, the camp was set a few miles off the state highway. We felt like we were leaving the "regular" world as we drove down a gravel road.

We went across railroad tracks, around a curve, and a beautiful vista of trees and open green space laid before us. Stopping at the main building, we got our cabin assignment. We headed down the gravel road to find the cabin we were assigned among twenty cabins dotting a hillside among majestic oak trees. We were ready for our new adventure.

We unloaded our belongings into our assigned cabin, including suitcases, bedding, and all the paraphernalia needed for Molly, two, and Rod, five months old. The cabin was a wooden structure with about ten bunk beds arranged around the perimeter. We had brought a baby carriage for Rod to sleep in. Molly could sleep on a lower bunk. Boyd selected an upper bunk, and I decided that I would sleep on a lower bunk in case the kids needed me during the night.

My mother and brother picked out their bunks, and we got settled. After enjoying a delicious dinner and meeting the rest of the families, we headed down to our cabin for the night. We settled into our bunks. As I was reading a magazine with a flashlight on my lower bunk, a mouse ran across the magazine. I made it from my bottom bunk to the top bunk without screaming and waking the kids, and I spent the rest of the week sleeping, fitfully, on a top bunk.

Even with the challenge of caring for young children in a camp setting, we had a wonderful week. In the mornings and evenings, organized activities were offered. After a delicious breakfast each morning, we had a time of family worship, and then we divided into age-level groups and enjoyed a time of study.

After our noontime meal, we would head down the hill to our cabin for naps. The pool would be open in the afternoons. There was a lake for fishing and hiking trails. During free time, there was always an impromptu volleyball game that Boyd and Rodney enjoyed. I liked visiting with the other mothers as our children played. Each evening, we'd participate in an all-camp activity, including a skit night, a night swim, and on Friday, our final night, a campfire. During that time, campers would share what the week meant to them and provide love and support to each other. Those campfires allowed time for reflection and renewal as we returned to our individual homes.

Family church camp become our family tradition. For the first week of August, we would go to camp. Everyone in our family looked forward to camp week. We attended that camp for ten years. Our life would have felt incomplete without our yearly retreat. Camp week was a meaningful restorative time for everyone. We found an opportunity to build close friendships with others who were seeking to grow in Christian faith and have family time apart from our normal environment. Because there was a strong core of ten to twelve families who returned every year, deep and lasting bonds developed among us. As the week unfolded, we ate meals together, played games, went swimming, talked, cried, and celebrated each other's lives. God's presence was with us and gave us a sense of safety and acceptance that allowed us to look at our own lives as well as supporting our friends' in their lives.

Each year, as we traveled to camp, the family topic of discussion focused on the big question: "Which cabin will we get assigned to?" This was important because there were no bathrooms in the cabins. All campers shared a ladies' bath/shower house and a men's bath/shower house located on the hillside among the cabins. I hated hiking to the bathroom in the middle of the night! One of my funniest memories was when our good friend Sarah was in the women's bathhouse and had taken out her false teeth to clean them. She terrified our little girls when she turned from the sink to greet them with her teeth still in the cup. They raced back to the cabin and giggled their way through the telling of their shocking experience.

As the kids grew older, they invited friends to come to camp with them. Molly invited her friend Mary Ellen. Mary Ellen's mother was very clear about how precious her daughter was and the importance of her entrusting Mary Ellen's care to us. Mary Ellen, like most kids, wanted to sleep on the top bunk, and I was worried she might fall out. We put three bunks together, shoving the third one next to the wall. I had Mary Ellen sleep in the third one next to the wall and put Molly in the middle. The final bunk was left empty on top, and I slept on the bottom—ready for anything that might befall us. After arranging the bunks, sleeping was uneventful; no children fell out of bunks. Mary Ellen was returned to her mother unscathed, returning to camp with us year after year.

The children played together, and shared in worship, meals, and games. Camp was the perfect place for kids to run and play. They loved swimming every afternoon as well as fishing in the small lake. When Molly was old enough to attend Girl Scouts camp, I realized that Rod would never be able to attend an all-kid's camp. He needed us to take care of his daily medical needs. I felt sad for him. He was growing up without knowing another person with cystic fibrosis.

In 1981, we knew that Rod's days were getting short. The August camp would likely be Rod's final camp. Rod was frail, yet he wanted to do all the things he always did. Boyd was recuperating from back surgery, so Rodney and I would carry Rod on our backs. Black eyes snapping, Rod was not to be stopped. Our friend Bill brought his telescope for nighttime stargazing. Bill enjoyed astronomy and told Rod a group of shooting stars was anticipated while we were at camp. On the last night of camp, we gathered on the hillside, hoping for a glimpse of one. Rod insisted he needed to see one, and as it got later and later, our prayers became increasingly fervent: "Please let Rod see a shooting star soon so we can go to bed!"

Rod's fragile health had galvanized my passion and determination to create a camp for children with cystic fibrosis. At the closing campfire, I shared with our camp family that Rod's days were numbered—and my goal was to start a camp for kids with cystic fibrosis in his memory. When we returned home, I began inquiring about how I could establish a memorial fund. What I could not do for Rod, I could do for others. Rod would leave a legacy.

CHAPTER 9

Rod's Final Days

When you go through deep waters, I will be with you.
—Isaiah 43:2

By 1981, the deterioration of Rod's health was dominant in our family life. Keeping the two girls' lives as normal as possible was very important to us. During the last year of Rod's life, he was often hospitalized, thereby creating a need for Molly and Melissa to stay with friends or family, which was never easy for two growing girls as they watched their parents and brother in crisis. Fortunately, my mother was retired and was a great help. With only a phone call from me, she would pack up and come to Peoria.

In June, Rod experienced his fifth lung collapse, and doctors were convinced that the end was near. However, this feisty little boy was not ready to leave this earth. Rod rallied and developed a bucket list of things to do. Coming home after a month in the hospital, he was ready to knock things off his list. We continued to embrace life with him. We carried a small emergency oxygen tank with us in case his lung collapsed again. He was able to walk only short distances. I often needed to carry him piggyback when he became short of breath.

One item on his list was golfing. Our minister, who was close to Rod, worked with the Peoria Park District to get a golf cart taken to the one course where children were allowed to play to give Rod a chance to try out his new child-sized clubs. Another wish was attending the Fourth of July fireworks show at Glen Oak Park. We went to the fireworks, but to my annoyance, Rod spent the whole night with my hands over his ears. Before it was over, he and I were sitting in the car. For Rod, sometimes the thought of the event was better than the actual event. Next on his list was attending the Heart of Illinois Fair. He wanted to see the grandstand show featuring Barbara Mandrell. Rod liked blondes. He enjoyed the fun of an overnight stay playing with our close friends at their farm. In August, our family attended the weeklong church family camp as was our tradition.

By September 1981, he was back in the hospital. One day, the activity director came into Rod's room. She wanted him to draw a poster for Love the Child week. He went to work creating a poster of rainbow with a pot of gold at the end. He added a slogan: "Put a rainbow in your heart. Love a child." Although I knew our time was limited, I didn't realize it was to be his last creative effort. After his death, one of the nurses shared her observation of the day Rod made the poster. She was amazed that a child as terribly sick as Rod was able to make a cheerful, hopeful poster. She felt he was unusual since most kids as sick as he was had a defeated and depressed attitude.

His days in the hospital continued with no improvement. One day, a dietician walked into his room. There was a package of Twizzlers on the dresser, and she proceeded to lecture him about not eating candy. I thought, *He is going to die soon. He can eat candy if he wants.* That incident changed things for me. I was done with the games. We were taking our son home to die in peace.

I listened to my heart, and my inner spirit gave me courage. I was tired. Rod wasn't going to get well. I didn't have a plan, and I didn't have credentials. I had a fierce mother's heart, fueled by the Holy Spirit. My heart was for Rod and for his two sisters who were suffering. No longer did Boyd and I have to manage life between hospital and home. No longer were Molly and Melissa staying elsewhere, afraid of what was happening with their brother. Our family was together, sleeping in our own beds, surrounded by the familiar, and supporting one another. We would face Rod's last week of life together. Rod came home from the hospital on September 11, his dad's thirty-fifth birthday. Melissa's birthday was September 22, and I prayed that her brother would not die on that day. Boyd continued his normal work schedule, spending time with Rod in the evening.

We were blessed with lots of wonderful people who provided food and support. My mother came to stay. During the day, she and I took care of Rod. At night, we would take turns sleeping on the cot in his room. A few hospital nurses who were close to him would visit. I was grateful for their presence and help. They would draw his blood or give injections, which, as a mom, I hated doing.

There was great satisfaction in being able to do comforting things for him like rubbing on lotion, bathing him, reading to him, or simply sitting with him while he dozed. Autumn was in its glory that final week at home. I recall having the windows open with a breeze gently blowing the curtains. I felt God's peace. I was not afraid.

Molly was in sixth grade, and Melissa was in first grade, and they attended school since we were trying to maintain as much normalcy as possible. In the afternoons, they would come into his room to report on their days. Molly would become anxious during the school day, so I got special permission for her to be allowed to call home.

I am thankful that I was given the strength to bring him home and take care of him. We had openly shared that he had come home to die. We were able to enjoy and provide the opportunity for our family and friends to drop by and see him. Always a social kid, he would insist that we took off his pajamas and put him in street clothes, and then we would carry him downstairs so they wouldn't be visiting with him in his bedroom. Ellen, a close friend, described her visit to me. Rod was dressed in his Chicago Bears shirt, looking very fragile as he leaned over on pillows to breathe easier, happy to be hosting company.

He gave exception to the nurses who had cared for him in the hospital. They could come upstairs to his room and see him in his pajamas.

A friend and I were visiting as Rod dozed, and she was talking about a Jell-O salad someone had brought when her mother died. It tasted terrible, but they keep putting it out at mealtime.

Rod raised his head and said, "Why didn't you flush it down the toilet?" Even in his weakened state, he still was Rod. He would have periods when he would struggle to breathe and would want the oxygen turned up higher. That wasn't possible since it could cause hallucinations. He would bug me about it. During his final afternoon, he went to the bathroom. I was watching him through a crack in the door. He grabbed the tank and turned it to see if I had it properly set. I laugh when I think about how he was always on. One nurse had a brother who played pickup games with the Bradley University basketball team. After seeing the Bradley basketball posters on his bedroom walls, she asked her brother to invite some of the players to visit him.

By September 17, Rod was struggling to breathe and was experiencing severe anxiety from oxygen deprivation. He asked, "When is this going to be over?"

I answered, "It will be over soon, and you will able to breathe."

That afternoon, I got a call from the Bradley University coach, Dick Versace, saying two players, "JJ" Mitchell Anderson and David Thirdkill, would be willing to come visit Rod. We decided on eight that evening. I remember telling this to Rod and then thinking, *He is so weak. I hope he'll be able to enjoy it.*

A little while later, Rod lost consciousness, and at five thirty in the afternoon, he died. His life completed: nine years, five months, and seventeen days. The sense of his soul soaring to heaven was felt deep in my heart. We were together: Boyd, my mother, my brother, and me. Molly and Melissa were playing with their friends across the street, and they soon joined us. We were together.

CHAPTER 10

Family Grief

Grief can't be shared. Everyone carries it alone,
his own burden, and his own way.
—Anne Morrow Lindbergh, *Dearly Beloved*

In *Dearly Beloved,* Anne Morrow Lindbergh captures the difficult task a family faces when one family member is gone. The grief is crushing, limiting the energy available for comforting each other. Boyd and I were challenged to support one another and our daughters. Ten years earlier, when our firstborn had died, I could avoid some of the heartache by changing my routine and circle of friends. I was able to work evenings and holidays when families would be celebrating. However, when Rod died, we had ten years of a life to honor and two young girls who shared in those memories. We had to step into the fire together and muddle our way through the grief journey.

Molly was eleven, and Melissa was six, when we embarked on the task of healing our family. Rod lived a full short life and left a wonderful legacy, but that did not negate the grief we experienced. Our family was forever changed. Just as my childhood was changed by my father's death, our daughters' lives were changed by their brother's death. That pain does not leave. The challenge of transforming ourselves into a four-person family instead of five was before us.

As we got into the car, Melissa would say, "There used to be five of us … now there are four." She wished that she could be a boy "so Dad would have someone."

Molly became a Bradley basketball fan and went to all the games with her dad. We stumbled along, each of us in our own way, and we slowly learned how to be a family again.

Both girls were aware Rod's life was ending. Molly could understand what was happening, but Melissa struggled with understanding. Before his death, she said, "Rod is going to die, and we're going to be sad and miss him and cry."

During the last week of Rod's life, Molly was more guarded with her emotions, and Melissa bounced in and out of Rod's room. Even with our preparation, she could not comprehend the pending event—and his actual passing hit her as a shocking blow. When a representative from the funeral home came, I sat in the rocker and held her in my arms as she wailed as her brother's body left.

School had started a month before Rod's death. His fourth grade class was next to Molly's sixth grade class. Soon after his death, we went to school for "back-to-school night." I realized Molly would have to walk by his classroom and see his friends for the remainder of the school year. I felt sad for her. Rod and Molly had sung in the children's choir at church. That year, Molly put on her choir robe while the one that had been her brother's hung in the closet, unused. My heart hurts when I remember.

Melissa expressed her emotions by writing over and over, "Rod died." In Sunday school, she drew a picture of him dead in his bed. She was open and matter-of-act as she dealt with her loss. Wearing his hand-me-down clothes and riding his bike brought her comfort. As much as I hated coming home to see his bike parked in the driveway, Melissa's need was more important than my discomfort.

Molly was quieter in her grief.

As I was driving, one of the girls said, "If I say something about Rod, will you cry?" I encouraged each girl to say what she wanted to say. I wanted them to understand that crying wasn't necessarily bad.

As Rod's birthday approached, I wanted to properly honor him and avoid a sad event. Rod had lived his life well, and I wanted to help the girls see him in a positive light. While shopping one day, Melissa wanted to buy Rod a birthday card and send it to heaven. It was only through God's grace that I didn't start sobbing.

On March 30, at the breakfast table, Melissa announced, "Today is Rod's birthday."

I explained to her that you do not celebrate birthdays after people die.

Undaunted, she answered, "He'd be ten, and tonight, we would have a cake—and he'd get the biggest piece." She concluded with her belief that he would have a cake in heaven and blow out the candles there.

I realized that I needed to make a plan to acknowledge Rod's birthday. I did not want the day to be filled with crying and sadness. I decided that Molly, Melissa, and I could take Rod's child-sized golf clubs and give them to the pastor who had taken Rod golfing. After school, Molly, Melissa, and I made our delivery and then stopped for ice cream. I didn't want to sit around the supper table missing him. We went out for supper, and when everyone went to bed, I was able check off one more first: I had survived.

Facing Christmas without Rod was daunting. One bright spot was a trip to cut down our tree. We got into the car and headed to the Christmas tree farm, our usual spot, only to learn that they were out of trees. We received vague directions to another possible farm for trees and drove away. Not long after we left, we found ourselves traveling down a gravel road that turned into one lane that was full of hills and curves.

We arrived at a crummy looking place with a crummy sign: "Christmas trees for sale." A shoddy-looking man gave us a saw and sent us off into the woods with the instructions to "top" a tree. We found a tree, and Melissa yelled, "Timber!" Boyd cut it down, and we cut off the top of the tree. We dragged it back to the car, lashed it on the roof of the station wagon, paid the man eight dollars, and went home. I couldn't force myself to use the usual decorations. The girls and I made new ones for the tree: paper chains, construction paper ornaments, and popcorn and cranberry garlands. We put the tree in the family room instead of the living room as we had in the past. The next year, it was back in the living room and has stayed there.

Traditionally, our family would travel to my mother's house in Farmington where we would eat Christmas dinner and do a gift exchange with Marylee and her family. That year, I didn't think I could survive watching my nephews open the same presents that Rod would have enjoyed. Unknown to me, my sister felt guilt that she had her sons and I did not. We stayed home. Looking back, the best thing about our first Christmas without Rod was surviving the day. No one broke down sobbing. We had a meal and played games, and the day passed quietly.

There were times when Boyd and I found it difficult to share our feelings with each other. We would hesitate to speak about Rod, fearful that talking about him would create more pain.

About a month before Rod's death, we were sitting outside of the hospital when a truck carrying a burial vault went by. I asked the unspoken questions that had been on both our minds: "Where will we bury him? In Farmington—where our first son was buried—or someplace in Peoria where we now live? How do we want to honor him when he leaves this earth?"

Our final decision was to bury him in Farmington, on the small hillside where his brother and grandfather are. We do not go there often. We find it a comfort that he rests with other family.

CHAPTER 11

Grief Is Shared

What we have once enjoyed we can never lose.
All that we love deeply becomes a part of us.
—Helen Keller

Despite our deep personal grief, we were supported by many outside the family. I had several friends who were my lifelines. I am extremely thankful for Ellen for listening to and validating my pain and struggles. She lived in Chicago, which meant all those conversations were long distance. In the 1980s, AT&T was a monopoly, and rates for long-distance calls were very high. I told Boyd that it was cheaper than therapy, and he would respond that insurance paid for therapy. We kept talking. Ellen gave me the greatest gift for a person grieving. She loved me and listened to me.

Relationships with our friends and family had to be redefined. The relationships lasted when we shared the grief journey. With some friends, it was too hard to move through the grief together to redefine our friendship.

One day, Rod's best friend's mother called to ask to borrow a Halloween costume that I had made and Rod had worn. I was horrified. The thought of anyone walking around in an item of Rod's broke my heart. I thought I would not be able to stand it. I refused. Years later, I recognize the request might have allowed Rod's friend to feel closer to him. At the time, I could only see my personal pain. What comforts or doesn't comfort is very individualized, and I try to remember that each time I encounter someone who is grieving. The best gift is to be allowed to work through grief in your own way and in your own time.

Boyd had to go to work every day regardless of his personal struggles. Many people ignored him because they were unable to validate what he was experiencing. In 1981, fathers were supposed to "suck it up." Family leave and the idea that he might need time off weren't part of the business culture. He worked the day Rod died, and five days later, he was back at work. Fortunately, he had a couple of coworkers who would listen to him and acknowledge his pain.

Nine months after Rod's death, someone asked, "Do you still miss him? I notice a hole there."

I was shocked. I was still trying to get through the day without sobbing.

For the rest of my life, I have to answer the question, "How many children do you have?" It's a difficult one for anyone who has had a child die. Do you answer the number of your living children? Do you answer the number of them all? Generally, I answer four: the number of my living children. If it is someone I think I will be having more contact with, I will add that I have two sons in heaven. We will always love, remember, and miss Boyd Dale and Rod.

Many years later, at Matthew's wedding, I was remembering all the fun times the cousins had shared. I looked at the wedding party and thought Rod should be there. Just this past Christmas, Molly brought us an ornament of a brown-skinned drummer boy that made her think of her brother, gone for more than thirty years. Many people who loved and knew Rod fumbled along with us on our grief journey. Many would join us in starting Rod's legacy of a cystic fibrosis camp.

While Boyd and I were dealing with Rod's health decline and our grief at his impending death, Marylee was also in a challenging period of her life. She had been diagnosed with scoliosis as a child. In recent years, Marylee had been contending with increasing back pain. The recommendation was to have surgery to install steel rods and fuse ten of the vertebrae. The surgery occurred in July 1981, just two months before Rod's death.

Each of us was muddling along with our individual challenges and struggles while desiring to support one another. In June, while Marylee was preparing for surgery, she would stop by the hospital to see Rod, who was recovering from a life-threatening crisis.

In July, during Marylee's hospitalization, I would go to the hospital each morning to see her while Boyd was home with Rod. Marylee, in a body cast and struggling to gain strength, felt the pain and grief of her nephew's decline and death in September. She felt her grief deeply. She had two sons who were healthy, and her sister did not. Marylee did not ask if either boy would like to see Rod one final time at the funeral home before the graveside services.

Matthew, who was Rod's age, was very disappointed that he didn't get to see his cousin one final time. Marylee was not aware of this missing closure for Matthew until years later, and she has always felt badly about the oversight. Through the writing of this book, Matthew and I have talked about his memories. Since Matthew lives in Farmington, he has taken extra care of Rod's grave. This has brought him comfort and created a special bond between us.

I believe the suffering of those times gave Marylee and me the momentum to invest in life, looking for the good to be derived out of the suffering.

CHAPTER 12

Fulfilling the Dream

Sometimes the smallest step in the right direction
Ends up being the biggest step of your life.
Tiptoe if you must, but take the step.
—Naeem Callaway

During the years immediately after Rod's death, Marylee and I did not spend a lot of time together. Our lives were more parallel than intertwined. Each of us had the task of adjusting to significant changes in our lives. I was dealing with the loss of Rod, the creation of CF Camp, and our eventual adoption of two more sons. Marylee was recouping her strength following her surgery and dealing with a failing marriage. Eventually divorcing, Marylee became a single mother, facing the challenge of finding full-time work and raising her two boys alone. She had great support from extended family, including our family and Bob's family. Her sons have grown into fine men. Life would change again, and ultimately, we would return to our closeness.

A year after Rod's death, Boyd and I adopted a month-old biracial baby boy, and we named him David Boyd. He was labeled high risk and eventually was diagnosed as minimally mentally impaired. David was a delightful baby and toddler who added a new dimension to our family. We delighted in the fun of watching him grow and develop; enjoying trips to the park and other kid activities allowed us to continue to heal. In 1989, we would complete our family with the addition of Geoffrey, age seven. Embracing the future was our focus as we continued to deal with the challenge of grief. Rod had lived his life with zest and courage, and I knew he would want me to move forward in life.

Before Rod's death, I was involved with the Cystic Fibrosis Foundation. Locally, I served on the board of directors for the Peoria chapter. The focus of the organization is to find a cure for cystic fibrosis. A cure was a priority for me; I wanted my child to live and flourish. In addition, I was interested in the aspects of daily living with cystic fibrosis. Our family was meeting the challenge of raising a child with this disease. We were interested in the insights of others who dealt with it.

In 1978, I attended a national meeting of the Cystic Fibrosis Foundation. One of the workshops I attended was a panel of young people who had cystic fibrosis. In the beginning of my journey of parenting a child with cystic fibrosis, I viewed the process only from the view of myself as a parent whose child was not going to survive to adulthood. As time went by, I realized that this was also Rod's journey—one he would travel without me. Seeing a group of teens and young adults telling their stories on the stage was a great encouragement. I was fascinated and inspired to hear about their challenges and ways of coping with CF. One young lady talked about her relationship with her parents. She felt protective of them and disliked it when she needed to tell them she was feeling ill. She didn't want to create anxiety or concern. The panel talked about the challenges of living in an unavoidable codependent relationship with their families due to their need for life-saving medical care. I learned about a new dynamic that would be part of the teenage years.

I identified with their stories and wished Rod could meet others living with cystic fibrosis. I thought of how nice it would be if he could know someone with CF. Because of our involvement with family camp, I thought a specialized camp would be wonderful opportunity for CF kids to meet each other and develop friendships.

When I returned to Peoria and suggested the idea of creating a camp for CF kids to the local board, I was told that camps and social events were not supported by the national organization. All monies were to be used to find a cure. Regardless, the seed had been planted in my heart. I believed there could be research as well as socialization and support.

After Rod's death, we established a memorial fund specifically earmarked to create a camp. The following year, we were ready to follow our dream of creating a Cystic Fibrosis Camp for other kids. Epworth Springs Camp, where we had attended family camp for the ten summers of Rod's life, was owned and operated by the United Methodist Church. They were willing to rent the use of the facility to us for our newly created venture. Close friends who loved Rod and had participated in family camp were ready to join our mission. We recruited both volunteers and campers through the local cystic fibrosis clinic that was part of Saint Francis Hospital in Peoria, Illinois. I was always looking for volunteers to staff the camp. A lot of the young energetic counselors came from my church. Again, God was laying down the pieces to make it happen.

We decided to start with a weekend retreat. In 1982, we had twelve CF kids join us at Epworth Springs. We enjoyed eating family-style meals, watching a twelve-millimeter movie, making a spice rope for our craft activity, and finishing the weekend with a group campfire. The kids thoroughly enjoyed getting to know one another. The weekend was a success. We were able to test our plan to accommodate the medical needs of the campers and provide the fun of being at camp.

After the weekend concluded, we felt we were ready to move ahead with a full weeklong camp the following year. We knew we needed to develop a way of funding the camp once the memorial money was gone. We would be competing with other charities and needed a connection in the community.

Our connection came through the Bradley University basketball program and Dick Versace. Even though the Bradley players didn't make it to our home the night Rod died, I wrote to Dick Versace, the head men's basketball coach. In my letter, I told him about our little Bradley fan who was cheering from heaven, and I thanked him for his willingness to send the players for a visit. Surprisingly, Dick contacted me and offered to start a running race to raise funds for our camp.

In 1982, we started the Race with Versace, a three-mile running race through downtown Peoria, led by Dick Versace and the Bradley University men's basketball team. This provided the funds and endorsement we needed to create the Cystic Fibrosis Camp Association that would sponsor the camp.

There were fifteen years of Cystic Fibrosis Camp to follow—all because a little boy embraced life fully and never stopped sharing his joy and legacy of fun.

CHAPTER 13

Cystic Fibrosis Camp Thrives

Still, what I want in my life is to be willing to be dazzled—
To cast aside the weight of facts, and maybe even,
To float a little above this difficult world.
—Mary Oliver

While researching this book, I asked past CF campers about their camp experiences and how the camp has affected them. I was surprised by the intensity of their feelings and the lasting effects after twenty years. The responses to my questions were heartfelt.

One young man stated, "Nothing else has had a bigger impact in my life." He was part of group of four guys who bonded in a deeply, caring friendship. Year after year, the foursome came to camp. They grew from little boys to young adults to men, remaining close until three of the four lost their battles with cystic fibrosis.

Susan, a CF camper, told me about taking her husband to visit the camp. She wanted him to see the place where she had experienced such great joy and happiness. When they got to the bottom of the large hill and were standing next to the lake, she turned to him and said, "You have to kiss me. This is the spot where kids came to kiss."

When we envisioned the camp, Boyd and I had no idea the lasting impact the week would have for the campers and volunteer counselors. The weeklong format for Cystic Fibrosis Camp evolved into seven days of fun and camaraderie while still providing the medical care the campers needed. We saw it as a service to a group of young people and a way of using our cystic fibrosis knowledge.

The first year, I was concerned it might be painful dealing with CF kids since my child had lost his fight with the disease. Would doing the therapy as I had done with Rod for many years be difficult? Would the pills, coughing, and other signs of the disease be hard to see? I hadn't needed to worry because I learned an important lesson: Rod, with his unique personality, was Rod. He was not a disease. Camp was a delightful group of kids—each with their own personalities—who happened to have cystic fibrosis.

Our first weeklong camp was held 1983. We modeled the week's schedule after the family camp schedule. We enjoyed games, crafts, ping-pong, volleyball, basketball, swimming, fishing, boating, and a campfire—all of the things one would expect in a camp setting. We ate in the dining room, sharing family-style meals. All the campers slept in two large dorm rooms—one for boys, one for girls. At the time, there was no air-conditioning—only large noisy fans that rattled all day and all night long. The original building was destroyed by fire in 1988 and was replaced with a new lodge with the motel-type rooms with private baths, air-conditioning, and a mezzanine where we could do therapy.

The two major areas of medical concern for an individual with cystic fibrosis are dietary and respiratory. Because the pancreas does not produce a digestive enzyme for fat, the kids were often underweight. Therefore, we offered three meals and three snacks a day. The cooks at camp coordinated with a dietician to develop our menus. One year, the dietician shared a bran muffin recipe with the cooks and suggested serving them for the midmorning snack. They were heavy as rocks and became a camp joke. Most years, someone said, "Remember the bran muffins?"

We conducted respiratory therapy for all campers twice a day. One of the main threats to the lives of those with cystic fibrosis is a sticky mucus that can clog the lungs and cause functional damage.

In addition, it often causes repeated bouts of pneumonia. Both of these factors can lead to death.

Respiratory therapy began with a medicated mist delivered through a nebulizer. The mist was inhaled into the lungs to thin the mucus. At home, they would have been sitting alone or with a parent. At camp, we had a room equipped with numerous tables, chairs, and aerosol machines. Each camper sat down and breathed the aerosol until the required amount was used. The room would become foggy before we were done, especially when the chatty ones kept taking the nebulizers out of their mouths to talk. Sitting with friends made therapy fun.

"Postural therapy" followed. Each person needed to be clapped (softly tapped with the hands cupped) on the chest in a series of physical positions, mainly with the head lower than the chest. Mattresses were collected, stacked, and arranged so we could get proper positioning for numerous kids at a time.

Each volunteer counselor would clap on a camper's chest. This was done as a group, in unison, with popular music playing and one counselor calling out the positions, timing, and running the music. As the music played, the kids would lie in a specific position, and counselors would clap on a specific area of their chests for two minutes. The campers would cough together, expectorate, reposition, and restart the process. At CF camp, therapy was the norm. Everyone did it.

Like any other youth camp, the kids would pick the cute high school and college volunteers first. I was part of the older crowd who were generally picked last.

Because therapy had to be done before breakfast, Boyd and I added a special touch. We would serve orange juice to the kids. Each of us took a stack of cups and a gallon jug of orange juice and went from bunk to bunk, awakening our campers. Sometimes we even greeted the early birds who had made it to the shower. The kids enjoyed this special touch; it was another way of making them feel special.

We wanted the kids to find all parts of CF camp fun and uplifting. The campers and counselors became buddies quickly. The campers' comfort in being cared for physically gave the opportunity to develop a feeling of intimacy. Caring relationships developed quickly. The campers found a group of peers who understood life with cystic fibrosis.

Jennifer tells of her first camp experience as a nine-year-old and seeing Mary, a camper in her teens, taking a handful of medications: "I saw Mary take her pills, telling me she did that every day, like me. It showed me I could be an adult someday too. I hadn't seen that anywhere else. It stuck with me."

Respiratory therapy was repeated in the evening: with all doing aerosol and all getting chest PT. Once a parent told me that her child fought therapy at home, but after attending camp, he had quit fighting about it and was cooperative. Occasionally, we would have a camper who needed extra therapy, and we would do that as well, always treating it as normal. Everyone took numerous pills at mealtime, another sign that they were alike in their need for medications.

The campers arrived on Sunday afternoon and went home on Saturday morning after breakfast. Because some campers came from out of state, this scheduling was convenient for the families transporting their kids.

The first year that Gerald attended, his mother could hardly bear to say goodbye. There were numerous goodbyes and hugs going back and forth until she finally got in the car and left. As the years progressed, his mother met someone and married, taking her honeymoon during camp week, knowing her son was in good hands.

After a few years of conducting the camp, we began to lose some of our campers to death. Boyd and I felt it was very important that we acknowledge their passing. We wanted the kids to know that they would never be forgotten. We constructed a special memorial garden at Epworth Springs Camp. On Sunday night, our programming for the week began camp with a brief memorial service. We would plant an item in the garden for each camper who had died during that year. Carrie had told her parents that she didn't want to be a plant, but she wanted to be a rock. There is a pink rock in the garden to represent Carrie.

Camp had become such an important and meaningful experience for the kids that some parents would travel to Epworth Springs to participate in the memorial service when their departed child was being honored. Kyle's dad came and shared how much his son enjoyed camp. The kids were able to share memories of Kyle with his dad as well. After the service was conducted and the missing members acknowledged, we could launch into our week of activities.

As the years progressed, annual activities became traditions. We always had a frog-catching contest and race on Tuesday morning. One of our volunteers, Bill, thinking with his engineer brain, decided since our camp was the first week of August, we could use the monthly first Tuesday ten o'clock siren test. At nine, everyone was released to go find a long-jumping frog, and the siren brought them back for the race at ten. We had a campfire and discovered the smoke aggravated the lungs, and the kids coughed a lot. The next year, Bill arrived with twinkling Christmas lights and "built" a fire using wood, burying the lights and cords so it twinkled and appeared to be a real fire.

Thursday was the obstacle course—a favorite of everyone. The Peoria firemen came to the camp to construct it. Using the pumper truck, they would make a mud pit as the final obstacle. The kids loved the mud pit. As director of the camp, I knew mudslinging would be part of the morning—and I would be a recipient. I learned to keep one set of clothes for mud pit day and would wear the stained clothes year after year. In another water game, the firemen would stretch a rope between two trees and hang an empty bucket in the center. Each team had a hose with a goal of moving the bucket to their opponent's end. How they loved spraying each other!

Evening activities included a skit night, a movie night, night swim, a hayrack ride, and a campfire. We were very open to tweaking the activities and schedule with input from the volunteers and campers. In one of the early years, the campers asked if we could have a Friday night dance. This became the highlight of the week. The kids looked forward to it, asking each other as dates, bringing special outfits, and getting someone to go to town to get flowers.

One year, when we had a camper on oxygen, they decorated the tank. Another year, a young man had fallen and injured his arm during the day. The nurse was concerned that he might have broken it, but he insisted he was fine—so he could participate in the dance. After he was picked up on Saturday morning, the broken bone was diagnosed, and he got a cast. My personal recollection was sitting outside the lodge, away from the loud music, totally exhausted, and watching the kids having a ball. Boyd and I felt a deep satisfaction in seeing the kids enjoying themselves.

Popular during free time were rowboats and paddleboats on the lake. They loved having these awful seaweed fights and would come back to the lodge stinking like rotten algae. I often wondered how their parents reacted when they arrived home from camp with a plastic bag holding stinky clothes. There was a pool for swimming, volleyball, bocce ball, croquet, crafts, and socializing.

We conducted all kinds of games, crafts, and activities to keep the week lively. The campers found peer support when the downtime allowed the opportunity for spontaneous conversations. I recall walking by a room and three teenage girls were chatting about the placement of a mediport (a device placed under the skin for IV medications) while wearing a prom dress. This was a safe and trusting community that understood. One camper said, "Camp brought a sense of belonging that was unmatched."

One day, when we were outside playing a group game gathered into a big circle, someone began coughing, choked, and vomited a little, which was not uncommon with CF. Without any fuss, we moved our circle over and continued with our activity. The feeling of normalcy and acceptance was, by far, the most far-reaching impact for the participants. At home, they were different, but at camp, they were like everyone else. The disease didn't need to be discussed because it was a common experience—a bond they all shared. Counselors were trained to treat the disease part of the camp experience as totally normal. No drama, no worry, and normalcy were the watchwords.

Each year, we would have different themes, and the theme was depicted on our T-shirts and executed in different ways. One year, we did a carnival/circus night with different acts. Megan dressed up in a ballerina costume and walked on a balance beam on the ground. She was our imagined high-wire act. Looking at the joy on her face was a blessing I carry in my heart today.

As the directors, Boyd and I always tried to do something crazy and fun. The year we had a carnival theme, we decided that Boyd could be the knife thrower and I would be his beautiful assistant. We upended a picnic table for the backdrop and dressed in costumes. Boyd wore a gold vest, and I wore a circular ruffled skirt; we entered with great flourish and drama. Boyd waved the golden knife around, promising a dangerous and outstanding act. As I leaned against the upended table, he circled to a bucket filled with water balloons, picked one up, and threw it. The balloon whizzed by my ear, and I screamed. He continued to throw balloons, and I continued to yell and duck until someone finally walked up and hit me in the face with a whipped cream pie. That shut me up, and everyone howled with laughter!

One summer, we used a holiday theme celebrating a different holiday each day. The day we celebrated Independence Day, we held a Fourth of July parade, complete with a cutout of then-President Bill Clinton riding on the golf cart as we threw candy.

Four boys shared a room every year and became very close. One boy's health had deteriorated, and he often struggled physically. To accommodate his needs, the group created a parade float that contained a platform with him in middle of it. The rest of the boys carried it in the procession. Their love, friendship, and devotion to each other lasted their lifetimes.

A forty-two-year-old former camper told me how she was profoundly encouraged when an adult with CF came as a counselor. "It was the first time I had met someone who had survived to adulthood. I saw I could possibly survive to adulthood, go to college, and plan a life." A college and law school graduate, today she is a mentor herself.

As Marylee's life changed with her sons maturing and creating their own lives, she agreed to come to camp lead the crafts area. Marylee, my mother, and my friend Judy stayed in a cabin together. Judy tells the story of the first year she came. Marylee and my mother were returning volunteers and brought little tables, lights, and other items to make their week of living in a rustic cabin as nice as they could. Rather than living out of a suitcase, Marylee had saved boxes to put her clothes in during the week. Using an empty top bunk, she had put boxes in a row, each appropriately labeled: Shorts, Tops, Accessories. Judy walked in and felt intimidated by Marylee's organization. By the next year, she had her own tables and organizing accessories. The three ladies were bitten by the camp bug and would share a cabin for several years.

Marylee was dating a man, John Nunley, and she would marry him in 1996. She invited him to come to camp. He fell in love with the kids, their courage, and their enthusiasm for life. He enjoyed watching them engage in all types of activities. John was originally scheduled to visit camp for a couple of days and then return to work. Once he had experienced the camp, he went home, asked for rest of the week off, and came back to camp. The campers had captured his heart, and he wanted to be part of the full week.

His experience was part of the seed that would become stroke camp. John focused on the kids, understood their struggles, and loved to see them having a good time. Today, when asked how he feels about stroke camp, he replies in his post stroke vernacular, "I like seeing all the people having a good time." He understood the struggle. He understood their needs. He loved seeing them interacting and enjoying themselves.

In 1995, MRSA, a new resistive bacteria, had made an impact on the lives of the cystic fibrosis patients. It became too risky to have the kids interacting and sharing rooms, and we were forced to discontinue Cystic Fibrosis Camp.

We grieved the loss of the relationships, joy, laughter, fun, and love of the marvelous times we had. Disappointed by this abrupt ending, Boyd and I accepted the inevitability. Along with other volunteers, we mourned the loss of an important passion in our lives. Not knowing that this passion would be resurrected nine years later and grow into a national nonprofit organization offering Retreat & Refresh Stroke Camps around the country. We trusted in God's provisions and discovered another opportunity where our love for people and camps could continue to change lives.

CHAPTER 14

John's Stroke

Often miracles are born out of heartbreak.
—Willa Cather

On a beautiful fall Sunday at 2:42 p.m., life as Marylee and John knew it was over. Two days before the national tragedy of 9/11, John suffered a major stroke. Together, Marylee and John would be traveling down a difficult road. It would eventually create a ministry to hundreds and a future life filled with adventures. The journey began with a period of loss, pain, and struggle.

Marylee does not know why she recognized that John was experiencing a stroke, but she did. She calmly told him that she thought he was having a stroke and that she was calling 911. They were in the emergency room within twenty minutes. After a flurry of activity, it was confirmed that he had experienced a stroke and was admitted to the hospital.

The first few weeks were a blur. John had experienced a left-sided stroke, which translated into right-sided weakness and a loss of the ability to speak (aphasia). John was confused, agitated, and unable to speak or communicate his needs. On the third day, John became angry and said, "This is bullshit." Marylee was thrilled that his ability to speak was returning, but it was an involuntary response, and he had not gained the ability to speak.

John had a history of medical problems, including a heart attack and two other life-threatening illnesses. Relying on that frame of reference, Marylee believed John would return to his former self. She knew rehab and recovery were needed, yet she held the belief that normalcy would return. Stroke is a different creature. While there was a definite beginning, the rehabilitation process continues for the rest of the survivor's life. Rehab is a long, drawn-out process with many failures and gains. The ongoing challenges can be frustrating and depressing. Recovery from an injury to the brain is different than any other part of the body. The healing of the brain is slower.

After numerous evaluations, his medical team developed a plan to address his needs and identify his rehabilitation goals. Marylee was excited. They were finally going to get started on the road to recovery so their life could return to normal.

A few days later, she accompanied John to his first speech therapy session. She was ready to support him as he began the journey. His first session remains vivid in Marylee's mind.

The speech therapist produced some cards with simple pictures. She would show a card to John for him to identify, and he would babble a nonword response.

The first was a picture of a table. John responded with some sound that wasn't at all like a word, and he smiled to see if he was right.

The therapist calmly said, "Table," and John obediently babbled another nonword.

As they worked through the stack of pictures, Marylee felt increasingly embarrassed. She was concerned that the therapist would not understand that John was intelligent.

In physical therapy, he needed to relearn how to walk. A common problem after stroke is sensory deficiencies. John was unable to feel his right side or leg. He was taught how to walk as they teach amputees: by watching his leg since he could no longer feel when his foot touched the floor. He has not recovered full feeling in his right side, but he has learned to compensate for the loss. In occupational therapy, he had to relearn the basic tasks of living, including the simple tasks of brushing his teeth and using the correct eating utensil. The amount of relearning he required was overwhelming.

Family and friends rallied around John and Marylee, providing support during those early days of crisis and rehabilitation. Four weeks after the stroke, terrified, determined, and hopeful, Marylee brought John home from the hospital. They began the challenge of John relearning the tasks of daily living. He didn't know what to do with the soap when he got into the shower, and he didn't remember how to shave. He didn't know whether to use a spoon, a knife, or a fork. He did not regain the ability to say Marylee's name until a year after his stroke. That first year, he would call her "my woman." Together they persevered in the slow process of recovery and adjustments. The first year was filled with appointments, and the demanding process of John relearning all the tasks of daily living as well as his ability to speak.

Many months into his recovery, Marylee's understanding deepened. She realized John would never regain all he knew or be able to do all the tasks he did before the stroke. Their life had become isolated and lonely. After working all day, she would come home to a husband who was frustrated with his ability to function and who needed attention after spending the day alone.

John was compulsive before the stroke, and this personality characteristic was magnified following the stroke. While he had always been picky—he was now very picky. More than once, Marylee came home from work to find a closet emptied onto the bed or table. John would order her to get rid of the stuff she didn't need. John had a need to get everything in order, whether it was a reasonable or convenient time for Marylee. When she tried to talk to him about his behavior, he didn't understand. In that moment of discovery, Marylee realized this was her "new normal." Stroke was going to go on for the rest of their lives. John was not going to be able to do the things a husband normally did: writing checks, helping with taxes, managing his insulin, or buying a gift or flowers for his wife.

While family and friends continued to support them, they were unable to fully identify with the challenges they faced. They didn't wake every day struggling to get simple life tasks done. John spent his days alone while Marylee was working. Marylee lived with the extra pressure of taking care of all the little and big things that John had handled. Their life was hard.

Just as Rod had felt the isolation of not knowing anyone else with cystic fibrosis, they felt the isolation of stroke. Their isolation over the next couple of years was remarkably parallel to the isolation Rod felt. Marylee and John began attending a local stroke survivor group. As much as Marylee loved the support group, she found it difficult to develop close friendships in just a couple hours a month.

In the past, gaining knowledge and understanding of the disease had helped Marylee cope. John's aphasia was their greatest challenge. His inability to express himself affected every part of their life. While she was researching possible therapies to treat his aphasia, she read an article in *Stroke Connection Magazine* about an aphasia camp in Oregon. The article sparked an idea. When Marylee had been part of Cystic Fibrosis Camp, she observed the great value for the CF kids to be together. Marylee remembered the fun, the laughter, and the warm, supportive bond that developed among the campers. She had an idea! Why not create a weekend retreat patterned after her former camp experiences? A place where both survivors and caregivers could find common support as well as the pleasure of getting away from the daily routine. This was the beginning of what would become Retreat & Refresh Stroke Camp.

Hungry for others to join her as she learned to live with stroke, Marylee decided to share her dream with Mary Kay Pilat, the social worker who coordinated the stroke support group.

Mary Kay embraced the idea and suggested Marylee bring her idea to the Central Illinois Stroke Council. The council supported her enthusiastically. Armed with the council's blessing, Marylee shared her vision with the Stroke Network, and it was met with overwhelming support by Dr. David Wang, medical director of the

Illinois Neurological Institute at OSF-Saint Francis Hospital and his team. Dr. Wang assured Marylee that he would find the money for that first camp.

With the Neurological Institute's support and suggestions for places in the community that might support such a venture, Marylee opened a checking account for Retreat & Refresh Stroke Camp. She applied for grants and looked for financial donations. Marylee invited Boyd and me to join her in the creation of the weekend retreat. We had a relationship with Living Springs Camp (formerly Epworth Springs Camp) where CF Camp had been held. Procuring the campsite was an easy task. An enthusiastic task force of volunteers with camp experience, medical experience treating stroke, and a desire to serve stroke families joined together provide the support Marylee needed to hold the first camp.

CHAPTER 15

Retreat & Refresh Stroke Camp

She believed she could, so she did.
—R. S. Grey

The name, Retreat & Refresh Stroke Camp, depicted Marylee's vision of an event that would include a mixture of education, socialization, support, and fun. She wanted the campers to enjoy the time apart from their everyday lives, offering the opportunity to refresh themselves. Marylee wanted to relieve her own personal hunger for support as she coped with her own struggles from living with stroke.

Much of her vision in the creation of the weekend retreat referenced her own experiences and those of her fellow support group friends. Her vision was clear: a weekend offering a balanced approach for both the survivor and caregiver. The survivors needed to be validated and supported—and so did the caregivers who had their own set of challenges. The survivors and caregivers attending would be required to be able to accomplish the activities of daily living without needing assistance from camp staff. Each set of campers would be provided a private room with a private bathroom.

Our task force of volunteers got busy giving Marylee the additional support and energy to execute the first weekend retreat. Walking back into the space filled with memories of our fabulous cystic fibrosis camp years we had experienced felt like a rebirth.

All the fun, energy, and good times were going to be recreated for stroke survivors and their caregivers. As with Cystic Fibrosis Camp, we would handle the stroke disability with grace and acceptance.

Our mission was to create a haven from the challenges of living with stroke. We had a vision for our campers:

Arriving at camp feeling anxious?
No problem … we will support and accept you.

Using a wheelchair?
No problem … we are ready.

Have aphasia?
No problem … we will wait for you as you try new avenues of communication.

Lonely?
No problem … we will interact, affirm, and engage with you.

Depressed?
No problem … we will make you laugh and give you a hug.

Feeling lost and alone?
No problem … we will provide acceptance and a listening ear.

Feeling overwhelmed with meal preparation?
No problem … we will provide meals and carry your tray.

Donna and Jeff were two of our first arrivals. The anxiety rose as they drove down the gravel road toward camp. Jeff was anxious and angry that Donna was "dragging" him to camp. Donna was nervous about Jeff's behavior. Marylee showed them to their private room, giving Donna a hug of encouragement.

The campers checked in and were settled in their rooms. The volunteers unloaded cars, delivered suitcases to rooms, and made beds.

After everyone arrived, we were ready for our first all-camp activity. Using a golf cart for survivors who found it difficult to walk, we made our way across a beautiful grass field, passing the swimming pool, basketball courts, and cabins, and arrived at a team-building course nestled in the woods.

The first challenge to our campers was for everyone to stand together on a wooden platform. With laughter, some struggle, encouragement, circling of arms, and holding on tight, the challenge was accomplished among happy shouts. Next was the balance beam. While standing on the beam, everyone was to make a line according to their shoe size without speaking to each other. With giggles and lots of finger counting, they completed the challenge. Through these activities, a community was being built. They were no longer strangers; they were people helping each other. No matter the disability as the survivors worked together, stroke faded—and the enjoyment of being with others replaced it. Everyone understood.

The weekend was designed to offer as many positive experiences as possible for both the survivor and caregiver. We were careful to tailor the activities to accommodate stroke disabilities, while not having stroke as the focus. We offered typical camp activities like skits, campfires, and even a hayrack ride.

Carol was a caregiver-camper, heavyset and short-legged, and she wanted to go on the hayrack ride. Unable to get up into the wagon, she turned to the volunteers and said, "Go ahead and put your hand on my bottom and push." She made it into the wagon and enjoyed the ride.

We wanted group interactions both in the form of small group discussions as well as group games and activities. Twice during the weekend, the survivors and caregivers separated into small groups, giving them the opportunity to relate to others who were facing similar challenges. They laughed and sometimes cried over their difficulties. Our campers had found a safe place to share their stories of living with stroke. Everyone enjoyed being free to be authentic. They needed validation.

One caregiver said, "This is where I am able to learn all the things they don't tell you at the doctor's office."

Touchy subjects were discussed like sex after stroke. The survivors found acceptance and encouragement in their group. If someone struggled to retrieve a word, everyone waited because they understood the challenge.

On Saturday morning, we took advantage of large gymnasium where campers could choose among a variety of activities offered, including manicures, chair massage, paraffin hand dips, and a craft of painting a ceramic plate. A speech and language therapist offered an opportunity for campers to try a computer program to help with aphasia. One end of the gymnasium had a climbing wall. The campers, both survivors and caregivers, got harnessed into climbing gear and challenged themselves. They were encouraged by the "you can do it" cries, photos were taken, and the sound of applause for their accomplishments.

For the people who loved being outdoors, a golf cart with a driver was available to transport campers around the facility. Planning for the survivors, we offered activities that had not been possible since the stroke. Adaptive fishing poles and golf clubs were available. We had several campers who were thrilled to be able to fish again. In later years, we acquired a pontoon boat, which made it possible for wheelchair-bound campers to go out on the small lake. The caregivers found time to relax, socialize, and share with other caregivers while volunteers were engaged with the survivors. Saturday night we had an all-camp luau with themed games. Judy enthusiastically participated in playing "pass the pineapple" and proudly took her pineapple home.

Volunteers came from all walks of life, including nurses, a social worker, physical therapists, and speech and language therapists. Some had previous camping experience, some had none, and there was a wonderful mix of personalities and talents. Everyone united to create a weekend of unforgettable memories and inspiration.

On Sunday, as Donna and Jeff prepared to go home, the anxiety and anger were gone. They had been replaced with joy and happy hearts. The two had found a haven of hope. There was no debate as the weekend ended.

We promised we'd return the next year.

CHAPTER 16

Stroke Camp Grows

There will always be a reason why you meet people. Either you need to change your life, or you're the one that'll change theirs.
—Loubis and Champagne

The first camp weekend had created a new community. I rediscovered the magic of camp, and others encountered the magic for the first time. When our team of volunteers left the camp facility on Sunday afternoon, we knew we had created a way to enhance the lives of stroke survivors and their caregivers. The leadership team was ready to plan for the following year. We felt our first weekend had been balanced with opportunities for people to enjoy themselves, get acquainted with others, and learn something new about their lives with stroke.

We had not had music at our first weekend camp. We missed it and envisioned someone playing the guitar around the campfire and possibly at mealtime. Marylee and I discussed finding someone to lead the music. God placed the right person in our path at the right time. My friend Susan, a talented musician, was completing her degree in music therapy. Susan had a lot more to offer to our campers than simply leading songs to sing. She brought her gift of making music, and—more important—she brought the knowledge and skill of using music in therapeutic ways with our campers.

I invited Susan to camp, and she enthusiastically agreed. Susan brought music therapy, a whole new discipline that provided a great enhancement for our campers. Music is therapeutic as it uses the brain in a different way from the spoken word. People with aphasia, who cannot speak, can sing. I recall Linda, who battled with aphasia, discovering that she was able to sing. It was the proverbial "light bulb moment." Joy and happiness flooded her face when she realized she could sing.

Susan suggested using a drum circle as our initial gathering event for the weekend. We opened our weekend retreat with drum circle. As we gathered for our first all-camp activity, everyone was invited to select a drum or a rhythm instrument, find a seat, and join the circle. I like to tell the story of Ann and Bob, her husband survivor. I knew from the moment they walked in the door that she, the caregiver, was happy to be here, and he was not. As we gathered for the opening drum circle, everyone was invited to select an instrument, and Ann offered one to Bob. He absolutely refused to take anything. Observing this from the sidelines, I grabbed a pair of maracas and offered them to him. He politely took them from me. As we began playing, he joined in, smiling as he shook them—success!

Drum circles have several purposes. They build community, create energy, and trigger smiles. As we go around the circle sharing our names, our weekend begins. Sitting around the circle, everyone is equal. Survivors and caregivers can look across the circle and see others whose lives have also been turned upside down. Led by a music therapist, the drum circle creates a rhythmic entrainment experience, which means the full circle is playing in varying rhythmic patterns. Therapeutically, rhythmic patterns activate the brain and motor neurons, often bypassing the damaged part of the brain in stroke survivors. This experience increases attention and listening skills. Socially, it creates unity and increases energy that enhances the connection of everyone in the circle. It is the perfect experience to start the weekend.

Creating a drum circle requires an array of drums and other percussive instruments, but Retreat & Refresh Stroke Camp did not have instruments and we were unable to purchase a full array of instruments. We were fortunate that Susan was employed by Illinois State University, and they generously loaned us the instruments. Susan would transport all of them to camp and return them to the school at the conclusion of the weekend. Today, we own a wonderful array of instruments, and returning campers have their favorites. As everyone makes their selections, I enjoy watching our campers decide what to play. Some immediately choose a big drum, and others like shakers or bells. Some even try several instruments before settling on one.

Since Susan's arrival at the second camp weekend, we always open and close camp with a drum circle. The sound and energy of the closing circle compared with the opening circle demonstrates the growth of the community that has occurred in the forty-eight-hour period. We sometimes have a camper who cannot tolerate the drumming, but no one is ever required to join an activity they are uncomfortable doing.

As we concluded our second weekend, we basked in the joy of bringing something wonderful to the brave people who live everyday coping with the difficult task of life with stroke. The planning team realized the development of Retreat & Refresh Stroke Camp was bigger than any of us had imagined. The campers embraced everything we offered.

At camp, stroke faded—and life was filled with joy, activities, and other campers who understood. The general public has little understanding of stroke and how it crushes both the survivors and caregivers, often leaving them living on the margins. There are many variations of the effect of stroke, and recovery varies with each person. Everyone's life is forever changed. Coming to camp changes their environment because they belong.

CHAPTER 17

Stroke Camp Thrives

People who are crazy enough to think they can
change the world are the ones who do.
—Rob Siltanen

The second year, Retreat & Refresh Stroke Camp held two camp weekends to serve the people interested in the experience. Our core team of volunteers recognized we had discovered a unique way to serve and support stroke survivors.

Marylee and I, along with other volunteers, discussed how to continue to offer the camp to a wider audience. We had uncovered a gaping hole in services for long-term stroke survivors.

Dr. David Wang, who had been part of the weekend, was enthusiastic and suggested that Marylee submit an article about the weekend to *Stroke Connection* magazine. Marylee agreed and was amazed at the response to the article. Survivors and caregivers from nine states contacted her. They were interested in coming to camp. The third year, we had campers from three states fly or drive to Living Springs Camp in Lewistown, Illinois, to enjoy one of the four weekends we offered.

When insurance denied long-term therapy and doctors said improvement had plateaued, many families were isolated with little hope of normalcy. A new world opened up when they came to camp. They met people struggling with the same challenges. They met people who were still making gains. They met hope, love, and friendship. We were confident camp was an event that could encourage and serve many.

Thrilled with the success with each weekend—and recognizing the great need for services for stroke survivors—we discussed ways of using Living Springs Camp as a programming center and setting up ways to transport larger numbers to the camp. The idea seemed cumbersome and had many drawbacks. As we discussed possibilities, we envisioned taking our show on the road, a type of camp-in-a-box. This appeared to have real potential.

Marylee and I—and many of our volunteers—had jobs and were dedicating as much time and energy as we could. The basic model of the weekend had been developed, and we knew what programming worked. We understood the needs of the campers, both survivors and caregivers. We needed to develop a way to continue to grow so we could serve more people.

Once again, God placed a person in our path who could dedicate time to the growth and development of the organization. Larry Schaer, Marylee's former employer, approached her about getting involved in growing the stroke camp organization by using the take-it-on-the-road model. Larry was enamored with the appeal of the weekend and how rapidly the camps had grown. He knew we had a ministry ready to move to the next level.

Marylee looked at Larry Schaer and said, "Yes—let's go for it!"

The first step was developing a business plan. The model Larry and Marylee created has been proven very successful. Retreat & Refresh Camp would charge a fee to the hospital or interested group. For that fee, our organization would find and contract with a retreat facility, develop the weekend programming, handle registrations, and provide the core leadership to conduct the weekend retreat. The sponsor would recruit campers and volunteers to assist the Retreat & Refresh core leadership team.

After reading *Stroke Connection* article, Carol and Dan made the three-hour drive from the Chicago area to Living Springs. They fell in love with the event and wanted to find a way to bring the camp to the Chicago area.

The stroke coordinator from OSF-Saint Francis shared contacts and talked to everyone who would listen about the awesomeness of a stroke camp weekend. Her enthusiasm and referrals gave Marylee and Larry direction. Initially they concentrated on hospitals and communities that were within a four-hour drive of Peoria, Illinois.

The local stroke coordinator, who had participated in the first two camps, shared stories with other stroke coordinators in the state. She wanted to get the word out about the great success of a Retreat & Refresh Stroke Camp weekend, encouraging others to sponsor one in their region. The first location signed on to sponsor a camp was Iowa. Unfortunately, a flood caused the camp to be postponed, so the actual first on-the-road camp was held in the Chicago area. The next year, we were in Iowa and have continued going to that site for ten years. Saint John's Hospital in Springfield, Illinois, a ninety-mile drive, sponsored an early camp. Every camp has been met with great enthusiasm, and stories of healing and joy emanated from each weekend.

Maureen Mathews, an advanced practice nurse at OSF-Saint Francis in Peoria, was part of the first camp, and she was fascinated with the beneficial effects of camp on the participants. She developed a study concerning the positive effects of a stroke camp weekend. In 2010, she presented her study at the International Stroke Conference in San Antonio. Retreat & Refresh Stroke Camp had a booth. A group of volunteers provided drum circle demonstrations, inviting the attendees to submerge themselves in a "camp experience." Maureen's presentation and the investment of a booth and volunteers moved the organization to a new level. The interest of the attendees was beyond our wildest hopes. Retreat & Refresh Stroke grew by leaps and bounds.

CHAPTER 18

Stroke Camp:
A Blessing to Many

> Still, what I want in my life is to be willing to be
> dazzled—to cast aside the weight of facts and maybe
> even to float a little above this difficult world.
> —Mary Oliver

Today, as we travel around the country, we follow the basic weekend plan we developed back in 2004. A large cargo van, emblazoned with our name, arrives loaded with supplies and accompanied by a group of four or five volunteers who will provide leadership.

The final preparations begin when the local volunteers join us (including employees from the sponsoring hospital) and the van is unloaded. Supplies are staged in the meeting space, and labeled crates are stacked for a weekend of fun and friendship.

The excitement builds as our team unveils the weekend theme and schedule to the volunteers. Volunteer assignments are clarified, the space is organized, and rooms are assigned. The profiles of the campers are reviewed, including how many wheelchairs and how much adaptive equipment might be needed. These are details that are quietly handled since we want the weekends to have an aura of normalcy. Every room gets a theme-inspired name sign on the door. We are ready. How will the weekend unfold? When will those special teary-eyed moments happen? When will we dissolve into the hysterical laughter at a silly skit or crazy costume? What new skill will a returning survivor demonstrate? What songs will we sing? What games will we play? What crafts will we make? What conversations will touch our hearts?

When the campers begin pulling up in front of the main building, they are greeted by volunteers who unload their suitcases and accompany them into the building. Someone parks their cars, assists them to register, takes them to their rooms, and makes their beds. We want the campers to feel special from the moment they arrive.

A first-time camper told the story of arriving at camp to register, unsure about participating. He planned on hanging back and checking it out, ready to make an exit if he didn't like it. He was surprised at the immediate hugs, hellos, and "So glad you're here" and "Let me introduce you." He enjoyed his weekend greatly and has returned year after year.

Our camp season lasts from March to November. We have assorted teams of three to six people traveling to locations in more than twenty states. The organization will lead over thirty camps, providing fun and fellowship to more than a thousand survivors and caregivers. Each year, the programming is built around a specific theme using a standard schedule for the weekend. While each camp is unique in the setting and participants, every camp will enjoy the same programming.

All weekend camps open with a drum circle followed with our first break-out groups. After Friday night's dinner, we have team games. The teams are balanced with survivors, caregivers, volunteers. We assign family members to different teams. We mix the survivors according to needs, so no team has all the wheelchairs or all the members who struggle with aphasia. As with all our programming, this is done without any fanfare. There are several events through the weekend that will use the teams.

On Friday night, our goal is to get everyone engaged in the game, such as music bingo with a giant card for each team or a relay dressing in a costume depicting the year's theme. The year we had a cowboy theme, there were mustaches for each person to wear. I discovered that everyone loves stick-on mustaches. They stuck them on their upper lips—and they used the extras as whiskers and eyebrows. What fun!

An important part of the weekend is the break-out groups. The groups are separated into one for survivors and one for caregivers. They meet three different times during the weekend. Led by trained staff, everyone enjoys the safety of saying whatever they choose, knowing it will be held in confidence. This is a time to share ideas and ways they have developed to overcome the challenges in their lives. Discouragement and isolation lessen with the knowledge that others struggle too. Campers support one another.

Saturday morning is pampering: paraffin hand dips, manicures, chair massages, crafts, and activities that are specific to the facility like swimming, fishing, rock climbing, boating, and golf cart rides. In the afternoon, there is a movie—complete with popcorn and movie theater candy. A caregiver exclaimed her happiness at being able to sit down and watch a full-length movie. She hadn't watched a movie since her husband's stroke. At camp, there were activities for him, which allowed her an enjoyable block of "me time."

Saturday night allows everyone a moment to shine with a theme-based program, including the opportunity for karaoke and dancing. The evening concludes with bingo. The winners receive fabulous prizes like flyswatters, back scratchers, lip balm, or pot holders. On Sunday morning, a worship service is followed by our final weekend team competition of Minute to Win It games and a closing drum circle. There are plenty of hugs, tears, and promises of "see you next year" as everyone says goodbye after Sunday dinner.

As we depart from each venue, we leave a newly formed community of survivors and caregivers. Relationships that were made during the camp weekend can flourish during the rest of the year. In some locations, tone chime choirs have been developed after enjoying the experience of using chimes at camp. Former camp participants often band together to hold a fund-raiser to help sponsor future camps.

At a recent potluck dinner for a group of survivors and caregivers, a caregiver looked around the group and said, "Everyone here has shed tears and faced the fear of being told your loved one has had a stroke. It is a comfort to look across the table and know that someone really understands."

Our campers agree. They wouldn't have chosen to be in this stroke camp community, yet everyone is thankful to have each other.

CHAPTER 19

Magic and Miracles

Just be yourself. Let people see the real, imperfect, flawed, quirky, weird, beautiful, magical person that you are.
—Mandy Hale

1: The Sisters

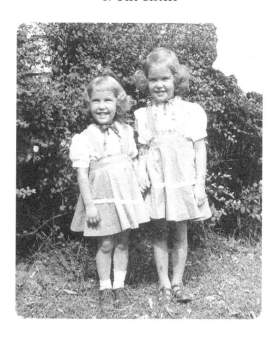

Throughout our lives, Marylee and I did not have a larger plan or goal. We matured, found our dreams, and used our experiences, allowing each to build on the other as the weeks, months, and years went by. We looked for God's hand in our lives. We learned and worked together to develop our mission by leaning into our passion and calling to serve others.

My deep desire has been to understand and share the phenomenon of the special experience of camp. I want to encourage others to continue to go forward in times of struggle and look for the good. We found the good in an unlikely way, and we continue to embrace each day looking forward.

I was surprised at the similarity of stories as I began interviewing former and present campers. Both Cystic Fibrosis Camp participants and Retreat & Refresh Stroke Camp participants told me about the special memories and experiences. I saw the magic created and miracles that happened, but I still wanted a better understanding of the process. The common thread through all of the camping experiences is the desire to be seen as the unique person God created and to feel validated as the real you, the hilarious you, the quirky you, the scared you, and the you who needs love and affirmation. Volunteers and campers alike need all those things and the magic and miracles arrive when we join together, leave our everyday lives, and experience "camp."

2: The Beginning Seed

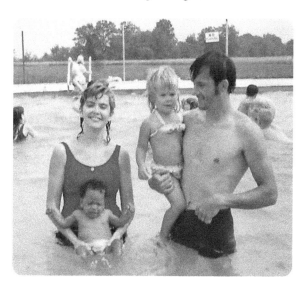

Our family loved our first week of family camp. We were young and full of hope. By the next year's camp, we had received the devastating news that our son had an incurable disease. During the ten years we attended family camp, our magic was the ability to experience a happy week together. Based on faith, we found comfort and support. Rod's happy, strong, mischievous personality did not allow any of us to ponder the sadness. Rod embraced the good, encouraging us to have a bigger dream: the creation of a camp for kids with cystic fibrosis.

3: God's Provision

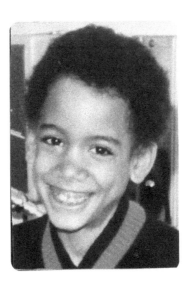

Rod's lung collapsed in May 1981, and he was rushed to the hospital. In the ICU, we were told that they did not think he would survive more than another forty-eight hours. We were surrounded by many wonderful friends from different faith roots, all praying for Rod and his survival.

Rod's uncle put his name on a Christian radio station's prayer list, and soon the walls in his room were plastered with get-well cards from strangers.

I cried a lot, sometimes carrying my tissue box with me. I wished I could "rise up on eagle's wings, to run and not grow weary" (Isaiah 40:31). I didn't feel like I was rising or running, but I did survive, always focusing on my family and my deep love for Jesus Christ and believing I was doing what I was called to do. I have held the belief that God could have taken Rod during that crisis in June.

Our miracle: God gave us three more months of life with Rod, and during this time, he completed his bucket list. Boyd and I became certain that the perfect memorial to Rod would be starting a camp for kids with cystic fibrosis.

4: Cystic Fibrosis Kids

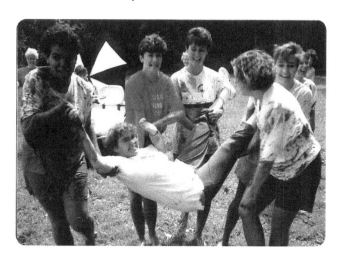

A collage of photos was presented to Boyd and me on the tenth anniversary of Cystic Fibrosis Camp. The photos are amazing. In one picture, Jennifer and Aaron are kneeling in front of the fireplace with their fishing poles and tackle boxes, ready for a trip down the hill to fish. Aaron lost his battle with CF, but Jennifer has survived, becoming a lawyer for the state of Indiana. She has experienced two lung transplants and is living her life to the fullest. What an inspiration!

Many pictures show the love and friendship we enjoyed. Blonde-headed Samantha is sitting in the sunshine with Joanie. Arms around her, the glow of the love of friendship and the joy of being together at camp shine on their faces.

Abbey is sitting on Judy's lap and getting a back rub, and Andrea is next to them. Deb is smiling from the side of the pool. In another, Jesse is sitting in the swimming pool with his oxygen tank on the side.

Jason, Chad, Gerald, and Chris are standing in the sunshine—covered in mud. Diane is doing therapy as Daphne keeps her company. Raleigh is holding a fish he caught. Shauna and Daphne are wrapped together in a beach towel. Three little boys are eating watermelon, and a group is playing shut the box.

In another picture, Bob is holding a spoon in his mouth, egg balanced on the spoon, and ready for a relay race. Bob was Bobby for many years, and then one year, he arrived at camp driving his own car and informing us that he would now be "Bob." Our golf cart is in the background of Bob's picture. We owned a golf cart to transport kids who were unable to walk long distances. The cart drew kids to it like a bee to honey, always begging for rides when they should be walking.

Kids are dancing on Friday night, a decorated oxygen tank among the dancers. Those pictures show a week filled with the miraculous moments of camp. Cystic fibrosis has faded, and friendship and fun are in the forefront.

5: Courage

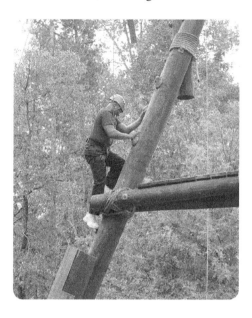

We are on the road to a camp in South Carolina. The sun is shining. We are in the beautiful Smoky Mountains. Philip, who lost his eyesight when he had a stroke, is ascending a fifty-five-foot climbing tower at Inspiration Hills Camp in Greenville. He slowly works his way up the tower, feeling each handhold and foothold. As Philip makes his methodical and awe-inspiring climb to the top, the shouts of "You can do it!" echoed around me. It is a magical and miraculous moment. We are encouraged by watching his determination to complete the task he has set for himself.

6: A Moment of Joy

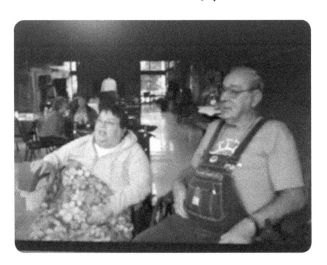

Our brother, Rodney, and his wife, Meme, were part of the volunteers who started camp. In retirement, they had become more involved in the mission of stroke camp. On February 14, 2008, Meme experienced a massive stroke. Poststroke, she suffered from aphasia. Her favorite words were "yes" or "no," and when she was agitated, it was "no, no, no," in quick succession and rising in volume. Meme received music therapy as the tool to help her learn to walk, to learn to speak, and to help with cognition. Most of all, singing brought her great pleasure.

Mel was a stroke survivor for many years and was confined to a wheelchair. A delightful person, his verbal communication was limited to "abba dabba" and "hot dog."

Meme and Mel met at a stroke camp. With the leadership of Susan, our camp music therapist, they provided us with a little concert of "Ain't She Sweet." As the group that had gathered around them applauded, both of them grinned and glowed. They had received the miraculous gift of being seen, heard, and appreciated.

7: Phoebe B. Beebe

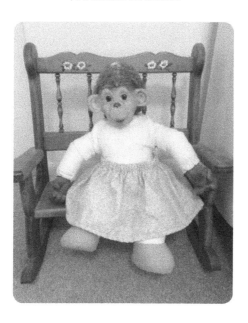

Phoebe B. Beebe was the doll who gave Marylee comfort during the grief of our father's death. Years later, I learned Phoebe cast her magic on Rod as well as Marylee. Unbeknownst to me, Marylee had retrieved her treasured Phoebe doll when Rod would visit:

> On Rod's visits, I would be nervous at the responsibility of doing his therapy. I decided to give him Phoebe B. Beebe to hold and play with while I did his treatment. Rod, with dancing eyes and a lively imagination, was like his aunt Marylee, a child of energy and creativity. Rod immediately loved Phoebe. We would play with the doll, enjoying precious time together. Phoebe was kept stored on the closet shelf, and she would come down for Rod when he came for a visit.

In the summer of 1981, Marylee made a trip to the hospital to see Rod. *I don't know what to take him,* she thought. *An inspiration! I will take Phoebe to keep him company.*

When Marylee walked into the hospital room, Rod—with tubes sticking out of his side—had his usual smile for his special aunt. He looked frail with his thin little legs dangling over the side of the bed. Her heart hurt for this child. She smiled, sat down next to Rod, and handed him Phoebe. They laughed as Marylee pulled on Rod's ears—and he mimicked Phoebe's monkey face.

Years later, our mother asked Marylee what happened to her Phoebe B. Beebe doll, and Marylee could not remember.

Boyd and I are moving. In preparation, I am cleaning the attic. Sitting in a corner was a pile of Rod's things, his leftover possessions I had been ignoring for years. I was puzzled why Marylee's old Phoebe B. Beebe doll in a brown paper sack would be among Rod's things. The doll was torn and old, and one hand was missing.

When I returned the doll to Marylee, I had no idea the depth of Marylee's feelings for her. She opened the bag, and the memories came flooding back of all the times the doll had served to hold someone close.

Eventually, the story of Phoebe and the healing power of this doll was pieced together. John knew nothing of Phoebe, but he learned the stories of how Phoebe became an item of love and comfort. He encouraged Marylee to embrace this memento from her life. Today, Phoebe has been restored and sits on a chair of honor in Marylee and John's home.

In 2005, Matt and his wife, Jennifer, had their first child. She is named Phoebe. For Marylee, there wasn't any name more precious. It reminds her to always look for the miracles and magic wherever you might find them.

8: Always the Encourager

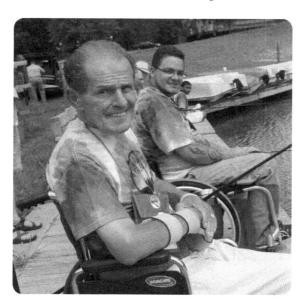

Larry, a stroke survivor, and his wife, Georgia, were part of the Peoria stroke support group and attended the first camp. Soon, they were volunteering to help at camps. Retreat & Refresh became their passion and purpose.

At the first camp, I had not spent much time with survivors, especially those who had aphasia, the inability to speak. Like many people, I would struggle with what to say and how to include someone who could not respond verbally.

Larry said only a few words, but he would not allow himself to be excluded. He taught all of us to relax, embrace a new way to participate, and not be dependent on only speaking words. A wheelchair was his main mode of transportation, and he would move around camp—with a little twinkle in his eye—always ready to engage with someone. He had little ring binder tucked beside him in his wheelchair with common words on the cards to help with communication. He showed them to me, pointing out one that listed a local bar. He was teasing me, which brought him great pleasure.

Larry's far-reaching gift was connecting with other campers, especially other survivors. As a survivor, Larry embraced life. He was willing to go wherever he could—restaurants, shows, and other events—not limiting himself because he was in a wheelchair. Other survivors found his zest for life inspirational. If a person was part of the survivor discussion group and talked too long, you could look over at Larry, and he would be gesturing with his hand to cut it off.

As the years went by, Larry began identifying a stroke survivor at each camp who he felt needed his encouragement. He purchased a special bracelet that said "stroke" and would give the bracelet to that person.

At a camp in Phoenix, a young survivor was struggling with accepting her limitations. When she began crying during group time, Larry went over and comforted her. When it came to living with stroke, the difference in age didn't matter. He understood and cared. For Larry, going to camp and reaching out to other survivors was magic, and he created miracles with his love and personality.

9: The Champions

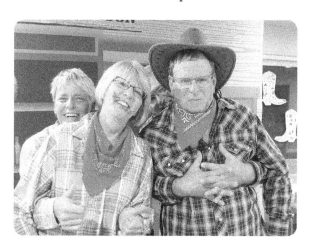

Successful camps need local champions working behind the scenes to bring stroke camps to their areas. I love meeting people who come to camp, fall in love with the campers, and become passionate about repeating the awesome experience year after year. Jan, Denise, Sally, the two Sues, Nicky, and Mary are some of the champions of Retreat & Refresh Stroke Camp at their hospitals.

Jan, from OSF-Saint Francis, Peoria, was at the very first camp. She had recently become the stroke coordinator, and Dr. Wang had made it clear that he expected her to attend the first weekend. While willing to go, she thought, *I am going to have to give up my weekend by attending.* Reluctantly, she packed her belongings and headed to camp. The weekend changed her. The way she viewed her job and her life was forever altered. She learned things about herself and her patients that changed her approach to her job. Forever transformed, she will always be her hospital's champion for Retreat & Refresh Stroke Camp.

Chris talked about her passion and desire to bring Retreat & Refresh Camp to her area. She stated, "If we can spend thousands of dollars on an MRI to diagnose the stroke, we should be able to spend money on a weekend retreat for the long-term survivor."

The Odessa, Texas, camp was started through Joan, a nonmedical person who had heard Larry singing the praises of camp. When relocating to Texas, she began working for a hospital and started pushing to bring a camp experience to Texas. A warm and supportive group was formed, and year after year, they have a stellar weekend experience and share their southern hospitality.

In Phoenix, the two Sues have provided the support and energy to create a strong stroke community that offers dance therapy, equine therapy, and a chime choir in addition to three camp weekends. Janice is in Boston, and Nicky is in Sioux City.

I could list the names of more and more of our champions from all around the country who passionately serve our campers. Their efforts enable everyone the opportunity to enjoy a weekend of fun and learning while we are inspired by our campers who teach us about courage and grit. These champions share the magic and create the miracles.

AFTERWORD

When I first started this book, I thought there would be a lot of information about the creation and the execution of a stroke camp weekend. As it evolved, I realized the story was about resilience and faith as Marylee and I lived our lives. My hope is to provide encouragement to you, the reader. In tragedy and bad times, keep going—better things will come. In good times, embrace the dreams and passions of your life—and always look to God for the magic and miracles. If you don't have a full, outlined plan, keep going. What is created might surprise you. Invest in yourself and your faith.

I was surprised at the lasting impact of Cystic Fibrosis Camp and what a terrific impact it had! I had great fun hearing the stories of our CF campers and counselors about the impact of camp and what they gained. The things they shared align with the stories of our stroke campers and volunteers: the long-lasting impact of the magic of being seen and validated, the relief of the isolation, and the connection with others living with the same challenges. At camp, cystic fibrosis or stroke fades into the background. We didn't understand the concept in the early planning. With Cystic Fibrosis Camp, my view was providing them enough fun memories to last a year while supporting their medical needs.

Marylee approached the creation of stroke camp a little differently. She was developing programming for adults, adding an educational component but still retaining the fun faction.

Ultimately, we found the same result. We were coming from a need for everyone to be seen as the unique individual they are. Every camp creates a community, based on acceptance, love, and validation of the individual and the struggles they face. For the kids, cystic fibrosis faded. For stroke survivors and caregivers, stroke fades—and each person is seen as a unique person.

Recently a camper said, "I can't believe the closeness and friendships that are created in forty-eight hours. On Sunday afternoon, you are hugging with tears in your eyes as you say goodbye."

As we prepare for publication, the 2018 Retreat & Refresh Camp season is concluding. The nonprofit organization will have conducted thirty camps in nineteen states, providing fun and fellowship for 1,200 campers.

There were many blessings along the way with the ultimate and amazing creation and growth of Retreat & Refresh Camp. From those beginnings, a recent new creation—United Stroke Alliance— has been formed. In addition to Retreat & Refresh Stroke Camps, the larger nationwide organization has a mission to educate the public about stroke through a youth education program involving classroom education geared to fifth grade students, as well as the BE-FASTER message.

BE-**FASTER!**

Don't wait, be *Be-Faster* to save someone's life

BALANCE — Sudden loss of balance

EYES — Sudden blurry or loss of vision

FACE — Sudden numbness, one side drooping - can you smile?

ARMS — Sudden weakness in arms - can you raise both?

SPEECH — Slurred or mumbling speech

TIME — CALL 911 NOW

EMERGENCY

RESPONSE — Get to the ER by ambulance, they know what to do FASTER!

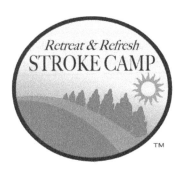

A Camping *Experience* for Stroke
Survivors & Their Caregivers

Every single day in the United States, approximately two thousand people suffer a stroke. More than two-thirds will survive, but they will experience a lifetime of recovery from the debilitating effects of a stroke. Of the approximate 750,000 people experiencing a stroke, only 20 percent arrive at the hospital early enough for effective treatment. Many are not as lucky and will spend months and years in their recovery journey. That is where Retreat & Refresh Stroke Camp enters!

Retreat & Refresh Stroke Camp focuses on four distinct areas of accomplishment at each weekend retreat: support, education, socialization, and relaxation. What's not to love about that?

A word that describes Retreat & Refresh Stroke Camp is *pioneering*—or, better yet, the phrase *a true pioneer spirit*. Isn't that what the heart of camping is all about? Getting out in the world and exploring new trails and adventures like the pioneers of olden days. Retreat & Refresh Stroke Camp is the ultimate experience in compassion for stroke survivors and their caregivers. It provides the universal need for a setting that gives survivors and caregivers an atmosphere of normalcy that has been sorely lacking in their everyday lives. It also gives those attending the courage and permission to be themselves and discover something new at the same time.

Nothing is more refreshing and invigorating than sharing the ordinary and extraordinary moments of life with loved ones and new friends who miraculously carry a key to open lonely hearts. Families need this comfortable and comforting setting to be freed from the isolation that stroke often brings in a world that doesn't like to slow down for someone who's walking or talking a little slower.

Stroke Camp feeds the souls of survivors and caregivers with compassion, companionship, laughter, music, crafts, and the old-fashioned spirit of camp. Retreat & Refresh knows how to do it right because we've stopped the world long enough to listen to survivors and caregivers.

Stroke Camp shows campers how to take back life. How refreshing and inspiring when couples suddenly fall in love again and dance for the first time since the stroke—or proudly sing for the first time after aphasia has robbed them of the ability to talk.

When the weekend ends, families take home memories, life lessons, love, and a greater appreciation of life because Stroke Camp reminds them how truly blessed they are.

Retreat & Refresh Stroke Camp
A Division of United Stroke Alliance
Strokecamp.org

ACKNOWLEDGMENTS

I am married to a wonderful man. Boyd loves unconditionally and has embraced my dreams. We have shared a life of ups and downs—always together. We're an awesome team. He encouraged me to follow my passion to share this story, especially when I was afraid to actually submit it for publication. The joke became that I would work on it until my death and then it could be published posthumously.

I have been greatly blessed to share this life with my sister: spending our retirement years together, running around the country, having fun, and using our natural gifts to create camp weekends. Marylee, you have always been ready to discuss ideas, words, chapters, memories, and perspectives. Thank you!

For our daughters, Molly and Melissa, I am very thankful for each of you. I am proud of the strong and loving women you have become. Thank you for your support in sharing the wonderful memories of your childhood with Rod and Cystic Fibrosis Camp.

Thank you, Carol Spayer. You told me that this was a story to be told and gave up many Monday afternoons to keep me on task in the beginning, convincing me I could write this. Your encouragement was priceless.

Thank you, Sue Mullen, a friend I met through writing, only to discover she is a stroke survivor and a passionate volunteer. Thanks for your writing skill and "eye." You were my grammar guru! See you at Panera!

Thank you, Phyllis Ackerman, a Bible study friend, who gave her time, talent, and advice when I needed it. Looking for a person with fresh eyes for my story, God said, "Ask Phyllis." I did, and our precious friendship was created.

Many others have been a part of this journey. Thank you for your love, your time, and your willingness to join me as I have lived my life.

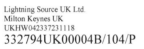